One Tiny Fault

An extraordinary ordinary life

ABIGAIL HALSTEAD

First Edition 2019

ISBN 9781709665394

PREFACE

It is important to state from the outset that I have been very blessed. I have been able to live a full life with higher education, work, good friends, supportive parents, a wonderful husband and three beautiful children. Not all CF sufferers are able to enjoy all, or even any, of these normal life experiences. My life with cystic fibrosis has, thus far, been relatively easy.

This is partially because I have always had excellent care from the cystic fibrosis teams who have looked after me, and partially because I have been fortunate enough to have never grown any of the nastier bugs. This is simply luck of the draw, not anything that I have done. It is also important to state that not everyone with cystic fibrosis has the same level of illness and I am fortunate enough to be on the milder end.

And so, I simply ask that as you read this book you bear in mind that this is not the life of a typical CF patient. The reality that most are living is far harder than anything I can claim to have ever experienced, or even begin to imagine.

For all CF patients and their families

-1-

THE BEGINNING

On a sunny day in April 2018 I sat gripping my nearly three-year-old son Ben tightly on my knee in a consulting room at our large local hospital. The doctor and nurse were trying to wrestle two sticky electrodes onto his arm, and I was both holding him still and trying to soothe him as he screamed. Eventually the nurse was victorious and the small machine on the desk started to work, sending a tiny electrical current through the pads. Ben began to relax as he realised that the little machine wasn't going to hurt him, and the nurse left to hunt out some toys for him to play with. The doctor stayed for a few more minutes to chat about why I wanted to subject my son to such an ordeal. We discussed his ongoing, phlegmy cough. For months I had been unable to sleep without having nightmares about it, but the doctor gently pointed out that Ben was a perfectly healthy weight, had developed normally in every way and was a very active child. It was much more likely that he had a lingering

5

cold, not a genetic life-limiting illness. However, he did understand my worries and why I was so desperate to rule cystic fibrosis out, despite my logical appreciation that he most likely did not have the disease.

Thirty minutes later the nurse returned and removed the electrodes. She carefully collected a sample of Ben's sweat from his reddened skin and left. Another nurse came and took a vial of blood from him, and with that we were on our way. Ben was pleased to be heading home, and I was keen to leave the hospital, hoping never to return to its paediatric department. Two days later the nurse phoned and informed me that Ben's sweat test had been negative. He did not have cystic fibrosis. A huge weight lifted from my shoulders and the panic in my stomach settled for the first time since Ben's birth. Ben had been put on breathing support for the first five days of his life after a complication during birth had temporarily damaged his lungs. I'd never quite got over the stress and shock of seeing my tiny new baby in an incubator with tubes everywhere, and a doctor telling me his chest appeared damaged and was most likely full of infection. Although the chances were almost impossibly low, the niggle in my mind that he had cystic fibrosis had grown over the nearly three years since his birth with every minor bit of constipation, tiny incident of diarrhoea and especially with any cold he caught. The whole time I knew I was being irrational, but finally I was able to see that my worries were just that. Unsubstantiated and unnecessary.

Back in 1995 my own parents had watched me go through exactly the same test. At the time I was a short, skinny, angry little girl with a sad face and distended stomach. By my second birthday I'd already had an operation to repair a rectal prolapse, the second in less than 12 months, caused by constant terrible diarrhoea. I had periods where I became listless and uncomm-unicative, simply lying on the floor or sofa and staring into the distance. Despite terrible bowels I was constantly ravenous; my tiny frame showing every bone pushing through my skin. My father nicknamed me "Ganny" after the seabird as a response to my seemingly endless food requirements. My parents struggled to keep me out of kitchen cupboards and on top of horrendous nappies (something my father occasionally reminds me were awful even now, 25 years later) and returned time and time again to the GP, certain I was not quite right.

Eventually, after 4 years of anguish, my parents took me to the school doctor for the routine starting school check-up. She listened carefully to their concerns and decided to find out what was wrong. Initially she tentatively suggested coeliac disease, and my parents cut gluten completely from my diet immediately. When we saw her again two weeks later she was unsurprised to see that I was still no better, and arranged an appointment for me at the paediatric department of the local hospital. She told my parents it was most likely either diabetes or cystic fibrosis and wished them all the best. The hospital doctor agreed with this supposition, testing for both in the same appointment.

A few days later, in the March of 1995, my parents received a phone call from the man who became my CF consultant. He informed them that their middle child and only daughter had been born with a genetic and life-limiting disease called cystic fibrosis. My parents rang my school and took me out for the day to the hospital, the first of many, many visits. I spent the whole day having tests and being introduced to a full team of medical staff – a dietitian, physiotherapists, nurses and my consultant. My parents were given a run-down of all the new medication and physiotherapy treatments I would need to begin, although to soften the blow my doctor only prescribed one medication to start with.

Naturally this news was a huge and devastating blow. Back in 1995 average life expectancy was 21, and my delayed diagnosis seemed likely to have lowered that. My parents were suddenly faced with having a child unlikely to reach adulthood, possibly not even seeing teenage years. It was presumed that the absence of any medication would have left my lungs damaged from untreated infections and that my intestines would have been badly scarred from four years of malnutrition.

Fortunately, despite my consultant's initial fears, I had somehow come unscathed through my first four years, harbouring no horrible infections in my undefended lungs. The enzymes I was prescribed enabled me to finally take fat and nutrition from my food. My bloated abdomen shrank and my ravenous appetite was abated. I smiled a lot more and became marginally less angry. And, most noticeably, I suddenly grew. I'd started my first year of Primary School as the smallest in the class by a long way, sticking out like an oddly shaped thumb amongst my peers. But I finished the summer term as the tallest. My feet, which had stayed the same tiny size for over two years, exploded in length faster than my mother could buy new shoes. Even my classmates noticed the change and I was nicknamed "the giant" for most of my time at primary school.

Parents of children with any sort of disability or medical condition are much more likely to split up than parents with healthy children, but good teamwork and understanding of how much strain the situation is putting on the other parent can help.

I was a difficult child and fiercely independent even before my diagnosis, but my parents weathered the storm and their marriage has survived through it all. When I had my first operation, aged nearly two, I was already so strong willed I fought the anaesthetist tooth and nail, eventually hanging off her head, my feet in the face mask she was trying to administer the anaesthetic through, screaming like a banshee. She retired hurt, and my father had to step in and do it for her. As an 8-year-old I was self-assured enough that I once wrote to the tooth fairy to demand a share of the profit after I accidentally knocked my brother's tooth out with a car door. Now, when I moan to my mother that my own children are hard work (and three in 17 months really is), my mother simply smiles and says "karma", so I suppose all has worked out in the end.

Although my strong sense of self was probably a burden to my parents, it has helped me handle my disease. Living with cystic fibrosis can be challenging. As a condition it is all encompassing, both physically and mentally. In a physical sense, it is present in most of the organs in my body and every day I must swallow vast numbers of pills, inhale several nebulisers and perform twice daily physiotherapy in order to stay as healthy as possible. Mentally it is almost even more exhausting as despite the endless physical effort that goes into staying well, CF is an almost entirely hidden disease. I'm constantly having to explain it to friends, acquaintances and the overly-friendly, cough-sweet-wielding stranger on the bus. Not many people have a full understanding of what CF is, and I'm always trying to find the right balance between being treated like a patient and being "normal" and fitting in.

On the outside, I look like anyone else. I'm admittedly a bit skinnier, and I cough more than the average person, but that's as far as it goes. No one treats me differently when they see me. But when I explain CF, people have a tendency to assume that the condition means that I am actually an invalid, completely incapacitated, and that I need everything doing for me. There are people with CF who are very, very seriously unwell, but I am not yet there. This is probably one of the reasons why awareness is so low. People don't appreciate how serious the condition is as those suffering from it are caught in a constant battle to live short lives to the full, whilst at the same time attempting to pop pills without judgement or the need to explain what is essentially a rather full on, initially disgusting disease to everyone they meet.

This may seem like an odd thing to a normal person, but sadly taking unusually large amounts of medication does come with a heavy stigma attached. The rudely healthy are always eager to pass comment on my pill habit, which is a constant source of irritation. It's not uncommon for a complete stranger to tell me to stop taking my pills, as they are what is making me ill. (I know. There are no words.) Even those who aren't handing out such insane advice are obviously made slightly uncomfortable when first faced with a person taking copious amounts of prescription meds, and well-intentioned "healthy" alternatives are regularly suggested to me.

I do appreciate that watching someone who looks so well swallow so many pills apparently at random during meals must be disconcerting. During rare dinner parties at university – always an attempt to prove we were actually civilised despite being students, our efforts always falling far short - I would casually take my large Creon capsules with sips of wine. Even people I spent a decent amount of time with would gasp and reach over to me. "Steady, don't mix medication and alcohol," they'd warn. Although genuine concern was being expressed it always made me bristle, but I'd always end up just smiling and saying, "it's fine, don't worry." Parties are never the time to sit someone down and explain exactly what's going on in my body, or even just why I can't eat unless I take my pills at the same time. Mucus and poo aren't the best conversation topics, especially at dinner parties, even if you are with students. But then when my friends and fellow students were fully sober and nursing sore heads the next day it never felt like the time to delve right into mucus filled lungs, or the nitty gritty of my flawed digestive system, so mostly explanations were left unsaid.

That being said, I have, to a point, always been open about my CF, telling people within the first few times I meet them. It's hard not to; within a few meetings even the politest person will feel compelled to mention my cough. And if I eat, well, that's game over. I don't really mind as I'm happy to do my bit to raise awareness, generally saying something like, "I'm fine thanks, it's not a cold, I actually have cystic fibrosis." This is usually received in one of three ways. Most commonly the commenter gives a brief smile and conversation moves on. This is person A, the person who has no idea what cystic fibrosis is, and doesn't want to be nosy. At the opposite extreme is person C, who knows EXACTLY what cystic fibrosis is. They generally look absolutely horrified and say something about how sorry they are, briefly asking if I'm doing well. Upon hearing all is going fine, they fix a slightly terrifying grin to their face and quickly move the conversation on. They will often furtively look me up and down with a slightly confused expression when they think I'm not watching. After all, I'm far too healthy looking to have such a hideous disease. This used to irritate me, but now I take it as the ultimate compliment. Person B is in the middle. They've often heard of cystic fibrosis but have never thought about it. They usually say something like, "Oh, have you? Isn't that the lung thing?" (or sometimes, much to my horror, "isn't that like mild asthma?") But the glossy, brief explanation I usually give is a quick thirty second overview with only a minor mention of mucus, and poo doesn't even get a look in. Bear in mind these conversations usually occur whilst I, and everyone around me, is eating. It goes something along the lines of: "it's a genetic disease I was born with, it means that I make too much mucus in my body and so I can't get the enzymes to my intestines so I can't digest fat properly. These pills are just enzymes to help this. And it blocks my lungs up so I cough a lot. But don't worry I'm really well, absolutely fine and you can't catch it." (A surprisingly large amount of people don't realise genetic diseases aren't infectious, so I add that in to reassure.) I've perfected it over the years, and usually that's that. Occasionally this conversation can take place in a less food orientated setting and I'll go a little bit more graphic, although this can sometimes back fire on me.

Once when working as a freelancer in a design studio an art worker I was getting quite friendly with turned to me and said: "So what, exactly, is cystic fibrosis?" I took my opportunity and began a full blow by blow account of exactly how my body produces too much mucus, and why this is a problem. I explained why I need to shift the stuff to stop infections growing, which will cause damage and also create even more mucus. I was getting into a real flow, explaining different types of lung infection and heading speedily down to the murky depths of the pancreas, intestines and bowel (in fairness she looked remarkably interested in what I was saying), when a fellow freelancer turned to me and told me how disgusting this story was and how repulsive they were finding it. At the time, I was 23 and the other freelancer was in their late 50s. When one's entire body is summed up as "disgusting" and "repulsive" it can be a knock to the confidence. Sadly, comments like this have been remarkably common throughout my life, and I've developed a rhino hide. Instead of retorting rudely, I shut up and coughed wetly at him for the next hour. Compared to the average CF patient, my cough is inoffensive and mostly dry, but it can always be amped up when necessary.

Now I will admit that there is a fine balance to be found. If a person wants to know details, but looks a bit weak stomached, I usually just talk about mucus as "secretions" which, although technically correct, is less gross but also less understandable. The problem with cystic fibrosis is that the bits that people generally tend to know about are actually some of the side effects and treatments. Lung infections and physiotherapy ("patting") are the most common things for people to have heard of. They are both correct, but are actually only part of a huge problem.

Cystic fibrosis is the result of mutations in a gene that manages how chloride, sodium and water are passed through epithelial cells. The epithelial cells are skin cells, and they are found all over the body. They are in the skin we have covering our bodies, and also in most of the tubes we have inside our bodies. Everybody has epithelial cells, and these cells contain a protein called the cystic fibrosis transmembrane conductance regulator (CFTR) protein. This protein allows chloride to pass through the cell wall. It then mixes with sodium on the other side and they form sodium chloride, AKA salt. This salt is important as it pulls water out of the cell, much like little salt gel packets found in packaging pull moisture away from the product. The water then mixes with mucus, making the mucus thin and easy to move. In a person with CF, the protein is faulty, and the chloride cannot pass through. As a result, salt is not formed where it should be. This means that water is not drawn out of the cell, and therefore the mucus in the tubes becomes thick and sticky. Over time the tubes block up with these sticky secretions. Or to put it better, they lime scale up like plumbing does in a hard water area.

So where are these tubes everyone has? The answer - all over the place. There are little ones in the pancreas and the liver. They're in the reproductive system. The intestines and nasal passageways actually are just tubes so at least they're not sneaky. And, of course, the lungs. If you imagine the inside of the lungs to be lots of little branches - well they're all tubes.

In a normal person, the CFTR protein in the epithelial cell of the lungs allows chloride to pass through, which mixes with sodium and other chemicals called mucins and creates mucus. This is normal, and highly important for keeping lungs moist and protected. Bacteria and viruses are trapped in the mucus, which is then carried up the wind pipe and passes into the oesophagus where it travels down to the stomach and is destroyed. I repeat. This is normal. You're doing it right now, and it's keeping your lungs happy and healthy. Just don't think about it for too long. Mucus, after all, is disgusting. However, in a cystic fibrosis patient such as myself, the mucus that is made is produced in copious amounts and is not like normal mucus at all. Instead it is a thick, sticky substance coloured from pale yellow to brown dependent upon infections. To be honest if you were to suddenly cough up something like cystic fibrosis mucus you would be at your GP pronto. It is so sticky that it cannot be gently wafted up and then down into the stomach. Instead it just sits. Obviously, this is less than ideal. No-one wants their airways to slowly close up because their own body is filling them with mucus. Therefore, we must shift the mucus by physiotherapy. This takes the form of exercise to get the lungs really working and then lots of special daily breathing exercises to shift the mucus up and cough it out. Children and teenagers are also patted to aid this, and I spent many hours as a child breathing whilst my parents took it in turns to beat me. Independent adults have to make do with special breathing techniques unless they are in the hospital with a handy physiotherapist to do the patting for them.

When I was first diagnosed my parents were given a reasonable sized foam wedge to put me on, head down, and pat me to try and get the mucus out. Every morning and afternoon before and after school I lay on my wedge and watched cartoons whilst this happened. A few years later, as I got taller, this was upgraded to a physiotherapy table (tipping table) that stood in my bedroom. The first time my parents put this up for me I made them rifle through the packaging and instructions to find a seat belt as the angle felt so extreme I was certain I was about to fall off headfirst. School friends often took turns lying on it when they came round for tea, giddily clinging on, and even in my university dorms other students would lie on it to experience the weird sensation. Like most things, after a few goes it became perfectly normal to spend 20 minutes twice a day lying upside down with my feet diagonally above my head and a parent patting me. So much so that I began reading a book as I breathed to help pass the time, my mother often nagging me to huff as I kept going with my deep breaths to avoid stopping before the end of the page. Physiotherapy is usually 10 deep breaths then 2 hard fast exhales or "huffs" to help move mucus up, then some coughing to try and get the mucus out. This is repeated twice on front, back, both sides and front with one side then the other slightly lifted by a pillow.

The only downside to all this physiotherapy, other than the sheer amount of time it took, came when the local paramedics visited our church youth group one Friday night to show us their ambulances and do a first aid demonstration. Near the end of his talk the chief paramedic produced a bottle of gas and air and asked if any of the girls would like to try it as, if any of us ever had a baby, we'd probably be given some. As the nearest girl, he passed it to me and casually said, "just take a few deep breaths to get a taste and then pass it on." This would have been fine, but at 14 I had spent 10 years doing 280 deep breaths a day, had a lung function of 110% and my physiotherapist often put her hands on the sides of my chest as I breathed in, telling me I had a whole four inches of expansion. It's fair to say I'd made breathing deeply into an art. I took my first deep breath, filling my lungs to capacity as I'd been so carefully taught, whilst the paramedic was still fiddling with the canister, so he didn't realise how literally I'd taken him. By half way through my second inhalation he was looking concerned and telling me to stop, then as I got into my third (by this point I was already quite high) he physically wrenched the tube from my hands, completely aghast. Gas and air, or nitrous oxide, is also known as 'laughing gas', and it certainly lived up to its name that night. I laughed and laughed, to the point where I actually became afraid that I would suffocate, I was so incapacitated by laughing that I couldn't even draw a breath. I was still laughing 30 minutes later when my Dad arrived to collect me from the rather sheepish paramedic, and the next morning my sides hurt from the strain. It's a shame it didn't have quite such a good effect during either of my labours, although the midwife did keep trying to take it away during my labour for Ben, joking I was breathing so deeply there'd be nothing left for any of the other women. Rather than laughing I hallucinated large angry sea birds, and the few gulps I got in during my labour for the twins simply lowered my inhibitions enough to squeeze my doctor's hand and ask him out for a drink; a bold move from a hugely pregnant, semi-naked, heavily bleeding woman who was clutching her slightly offended husband's arm with her other hand.

Unfortunately, even with daily physiotherapy, it's very difficult to get all of the mucus out, and so over time it builds up and cause problems. The presence of the mucus, combined with the effort to remove these build ups leads to swelling and inflammation in the tissue which doesn't help with lung function either. To add to this delightful mix, the special mucus that CF patients have is a perfect breeding ground for bacteria. This results in frequent and often long-lasting lung infections, which, in turn, produce more mucus and more inflammation. It's a vicious cycle that's almost impossible to break. The infections are caused by bacteria (bugs). These bugs are nasty things that turn up in the lungs unannounced and settle themselves into the perfect conditions provided by CF lungs. They then barricade themselves in by making little shields (biofilms) and start having wild parties, wrecking the joint and breeding all over the place.

In an attempt to stop these bugs, I take copious amounts of antibiotics. Some are prophylactic, which means that they are taken to help ward off the infections before they happen, and some are targeted. These are either pills, inhaled nebulisers, or IV drugs. At the same time as taking these antibiotics, I inhale medications through a nebuliser to help loosen the mucus up to help it be coughed out. All this is time consuming, and can often feel a little pointless. At first these medications have a small, measurable effect, but what they're really for is helping stop any problems before they become too big. It's cumulative and therefore difficult for me to exactly measure their value as it's stability and lack of deterioration that is usually being measured, as opposed to improvement. But they are doing a vital job, and not taking them would be a quick way to disaster. Although these drugs are all important and do help a lot, there is an inevitability to cystic fibrosis that can't be ignored. However hard a person tries to keep on top of the condition it will worsen with time and eventually it will win. The body is not designed to lime scale up in such a way, and even heavy routine maintenance will eventually not be enough.

Whilst regular treatments do help, there is also a heavy element of luck involved. In comparison to most CF patients I am well, but this is mostly because I have never grown any of the most horrendous bugs. There's no real reason for this as the bugs are everywhere – airborne, waterborne, on rotting vegetation... the list could go on. Yet somehow, I have gotten through 28 years dodging most. There is a common misconception that those who are very ill with their cystic fibrosis are ill because they haven't take care of themselves enough. An acquaintance of mine once told me about another CF patient she knew. The girl had been so unwell she needed a lung transplant in her early 20s. Rather than expressing sympathy, the woman said, "it's been horrible for her, but hopefully she'll look after these lungs more." I am grateful every day that I am nowhere near the transplant stage, but it horrifies me that reaching that stage could come with the idea that I'd somehow put myself in that position. No one wants to be ill, but sadly how ill a person becomes, and how fast that happens, is not really something anyone can control.

Having CF, I became accustomed from a very early age to taking a lot of pills and doing a lot of physio and exercise. To me my life is normal, although from the outside it may look anything but. Every now and again something happens that makes me realise just how strange my situation must seem to anyone not in the know. Having recently moved into a new stage of life in becoming a mother, I have met a lot of new people, and this has brought the oddness of my CF to the forefront.

My house, like I suppose all tiny houses inhabited by a multitude of miniature dictators, is a disaster zone. The mess is overwhelming, a slovenly chaos of toys, washing (who knows what's clean or dirty anymore, the piles mixed a long time ago, and I operate on a sniff test policy, shoving clothes at household members as they pass every morning), paperwork (both business and personal), dog toys, random screws and tools (a situation anyone living with a tradesperson will appreciate) and assorted pill bottles. Reading this you are probably appalled, but we are five people and a dog in a very small house with only a living-stroke-dining room, a little loo and a small kitchen downstairs. It's not a house we intended to have three children in, but as we never expected to have three children that's not really a surprise. Tidying, quite simply, is not high on my list of life's priorities. I wasn't exactly house proud before I had children, so the situation was never going to be great. I realised early on in the twins' life that the best thing to do was vacuum through the detritus every few days, thus giving the impression that the house is at least clean and that any surprise guest has just caught me in the middle of a good old sort out. Regular visitors are probably wise to this by now, but to be honest anyone who cares too much about how tidy my house is isn't really welcome anyway.

As for the medication bottles and medical paraphernalia littering the kitchen surfaces and general floor space, I decided from the very beginning that hiding medication from small children was not only impossible, but could actually be dangerous. To a toddler there is nothing more exciting than something they're not allowed to have, and my children are all extremely talented at stealing things they think might be interesting. My medication is, therefore, never hidden and in fact the children help me count my pills out every meal time. This, combined with the fact that I'm almost constantly eating, means that my house is littered with Creon pots. The children also often sit and watch me nebulise, or, as Ben likes to tell random adults, they sit and watch me "smoke my special medicine". They also enjoy taking it in turns to try breathing through my little physiotherapy aid, a small pipe like thing called an Aerobika. It goes without saying that they aren't allowed to do any of this unsupervised, and they know that the tablets are "Mummy's tablets" and not for them to touch or take. They're just not kept as some sort of forbidden fruit. The girls frequently tell me that when they are mummies themselves they will have their own tablets, but we'll cross that bridge when they're older.

As a result of all this, our chaotic house has become normal and I forget that to an outsider the juxtaposition of pills and toys is somewhat unsettling. I was made horribly aware of this once after one of the few times that my husband and I organised for a babysitter to come whilst we went out for a rare date night. The lady arrived at our house just after the children had gone to bed, and we settled her in, apologising profusely for the mess, whilst showing her where she could get refreshments and demonstrating the TV for her. We then left and had a lovely, quiet evening all to ourselves. Upon our return, we opened the door to a remarkably tidy living room, with the toys all either put away or neatly stacked. Surprised, and feeling that she had gone above and beyond her remit as babysitter, I thanked her and opened my purse to give her the prearranged sum of cash for her services, desperately searching for some sort of tip as well. Rather than take any of the money she shook her head and backed away towards the door. "Oh no, Mrs Halstead," she said, "there's no need to worry, this one's on me." I pressed the money on her again, but she refused and disappeared off out the door, briefly, but uncertainly, squeezing my hand before she left. Nonplussed I put the money back in my purse and looked at John. He shrugged and headed off to the kitchen. Before I could finish taking my coat off he called me over. I walked into our little kitchen to see the lady had not only washed up and cleaned the sides for us, but had also carefully collected and laid out every pill bottle, supplement and nebuliser part from around the downstairs of our house. Embarrassingly, she had also found not only the sharps bucket, but also a pack of sterile sealed needles, which she had laid on top of the bright yellow bin. Fortunately, all my meds are well labelled and obviously prescribed, but I do wonder what she thought was wrong with me as she unearthed more and more pots, and how serious she must have considered the situation to be that she had chosen to spend her entire evening cleaning for us. Shortly after this incident we set up a babysitting club with a group of parent friends, so I will never get the chance to ask her or explain. Although perhaps that's for the best.

Back in 1995 I was diagnosed with CF on a Friday. My parents had already arranged with family friends to meet up on the Saturday and visit a museum half way between our families. They phoned their friends on the Friday night to explain what had happened. Their friends were devastated for them, and offered to cancel the next day's excursion, presuming we would need time to process what had happened. My parents decided not to cancel, realising that life needed to go on as normal. I had been born with a condition, I would never get rid of it, but there was no need to live life any differently because of it. This profound moment set my life on a course from then on. I have tried to live a normal life every day since then. Yes, sometimes things are that bit harder, but I see my CF as just a side line to my life, not the main event. My parents never treated me any differently from my brothers unless they had to. I lived life with them normally; camping in summers, climbing mountains, playing out with friends. And, so far, I have lived the life that I want to lead.

-2-

SCHOOL

The time that I spent at school was a wonderfully happy time. I understand from my various forays into cystic fibrosis internet forums that bullying at school is a real issue, particularly for teenagers. The nature of CF means that even when we are younger we are intrinsically different from our peers. We are generally skinnier, paler and cough more than the people we hang round with, and that's without popping copious amounts of pills and vanishing off to hospital for weeks or even months at a time. A lot of more severely affected patients are also likely to suffer fatigue from the exhaustion of coughing their guts out all day and night, whilst simultaneously fighting deep rooted infections in their lungs and eating what feels like their own body weight in food every day at the same time. All of this, combined with the hidden nature of CF – after all what teenager wants to explain their digestive system doesn't work properly, or explain (yet again!) that yes, your parents beat you to help you cough out "snot" - makes social interactions at school a little challenging. This means patients often feel isolated, lonely and are an easy target for bullies at school. I understand from general internet chats that a lot hide their condition as well as they can, and have heard of teenagers becoming non-compliant with their meds in a desperate attempt to be more 'normal'. Obviously, this approach has serious consequences, and can be devastating in the long term.

Fortunately, I never had these problems. This was partly because my CF has been mild and I haven't (yet!) caught any of the nastier bugs, therefore I avoided IVs and hospital stays until my early 20s, meaning that I only missed school for routine appointments. It was also partly because my parents signed me up, aged seven, to a Judo club. For eleven years I spent several hours a week fighting people, which gave me enough self-confidence to tell my peers all about the gross world of CF whenever they mentioned it without any fear of them calling me names. Or at least not doing it to my face anyway.

Unusually I was also diagnosed after I'd already started reception, and as a result my school teachers learned about CF at the same rate as my parents, and were keen to support both me and my parents however they could. Almost overnight I went from odd-looking but generally normal school girl to a normal-looking heavy drug user.

My time in the infants came with a few privileges. My parents arranged with my head teacher that she would be in charge of my antibiotics, which were spooned into my mouth at the start of morning break time. This was seen by my class mates as something of a treat. I left the classroom just before everyone else every day, sat on her special comfy chair and came away with a mouth full of toffee from the bag she kept in her desk drawer to help take away the hideous "banana" flavoured flucloxacillin. Naturally I didn't tell my friends the medicine tasted disgusting; after all, why ruin the illusion? As for the rest of my medication, which at first was just Creon to replace absent pancreatic enzymes and the four different fat soluble vitamins my body was unable to absorb, I simply kept them in a pot in my lunchbox and took them myself. My mother, on the advice of my consultant, decided that the best way to help me swallow my Creon would be to break them open and mix the tiny pellets inside with jam. I would then eat a spoon full of jam periodically throughout a meal. This was a good idea and very effective, but also repulsive in both taste and texture beyond description. As a result, I learned to swallow very quickly. The school decided it would be best to assign a year 6 pupil to come and stand next to me in the canteen at dinner time and remind me to take my pills. The girl, whose name I sadly can't remember, did not know what was wrong with me and was only privy to the name of one of my more innocuous medications. "Don't forget your vitamin K, Abigail!"

She would enthusiastically shout in my ear every day, gleeful at the level of responsibility she had been given. I would duly take my tiny orange vitamin K, and she would vanish off to eat her own lunch, happy in the knowledge that her duty had been done. I would then proceed to take the remaining handful in one big gulp, much to the noisy awe and excitement of the other children on my table, in a five-year-olds equivalent of "Chug! Chug! Chug!" After a few months, the fights to sit on my table and watch this display, combined with my willingness to share my ridiculously huge lunch box stash of crisps and chocolate, led the teachers to threaten me that they would make me sit on their table at lunch if I didn't start taking my pills and condition more seriously. I complied, although even at university the party trick ability to dry swallow seven relatively large capsules caused merriment amongst fellow students. By the time I was in juniors, healthy eating initiatives had kicked in with a vengeance, and I found myself carrying a lunchbox full of coveted contraband to the canteen every day. This was fantastic for me, and I was happy to swap my fat filled, sugar coated treats for better seats in assembly, new fountain pens and the chance to feed the classroom pet on whichever days I wanted.

As I progressed through primary school my medication intake increased. I began taking supplements to help boost my weight (although in hindsight, if I'd been slightly less generous with my snacks, I might not have needed quite so many quite so early) and so I started having a daily Fortisip with my morning snack.

Gaining and maintaining weight is difficult for CF patients. Our bodies are constantly being put under pressure by the infections in our lungs, and we need a constant supply of calories in order to have the energy to fight them. As our pancreases don't work properly, we need to eat even more on top of this as we are not absorbing everything that we take in, and are unable to digest fat at all. My dietitian recently told me that it is believed that a CF patient requires approximately 200-300% of the calories that a normal person requires, just to live normally.

The ability to eat huge amounts of "bad" foods without adding inches to a waist band often seems like one of the only perks of having CF. When people (almost invariably female) comment on the food they see me eating they often express envy that I don't have to watch my weight at all, and that eating endless chocolate and chips is actually praised by my dietitian. Of course, just like anyone else I must eat the "healthy" bits as well as they are still important, although ideally CF patients should eat their vegetables smothered in butter and their fruit coated in cream. It sounds amazing, but believe me, there definitely can be too much of a good thing.

I never really appreciated just how much I need to eat compared to everyone else until I began to do the food shopping for myself. Before I discovered the wonders of online shopping, I would routinely have judgement passed on my trolley by the checkout assistant. At first, they would shake their heads slightly and tell me I'd never keep my figure if I ate like this. As I've gotten older and skinnier, people have commented that I'm probably not eating the right sort of food, or just looked at the amount, then at me, then back to the trolley slightly confused. They probably think I'm a feeder, as I couldn't possibly be so skinny and eat all that. I can't imagine what they'd say if they knew I was eating all that and cramming ridiculously high calorie supplements in at the same time.

In the 1990s Fortisip came in a tall juice box like carton, although now it comes in a little plastic bottle. It has the consistency of past it's best milk and was flavoured either chocolate, strawberry, banana or, interestingly, pineapple. This was outside the box, but not in a good way. Needless to say, these were absolutely hideous, but as they were very high in calories I held my nose and consumed one a day. That is until year 5, when I got cocky and began to hide them, very discreetly, in the bin. My teacher every year always made sure they gave it to me at the start of break time so I could drink it all in the playground, and then watched me bin it at the end. I, however, figured out that if I pushed the straw inside and tucked the end in too it wouldn't leak and I could just bin it at the end of break time without anyone knowing I'd never taken a sip. Although this may sound obvious to an adult, to a just turned nine-year-old this was a genius move that took nearly a week to perfect, and all my self-control not to show everyone. This worked for several months before the class bin somehow went through a half term holiday without being emptied. Needless to say, the stench of already smelly and now gone off Fortisip was vile and the classroom reeked. To make matters worse, the straw had become unstuck and my teacher was drenched in the Fortisip when he came in on the Monday morning and accidentally split the bag in his hurry to empty the bin and dispose of the smelly rubbish. In what I now see as a great example of calm self-control my teacher, rather than yell at me about his stinking ruined trousers, asked me to sit with him at break. We sat together on a table next to a radiator, his PE shorts clearly not as warm as his trousers, and talked about how horrible Fortisip was, but why it was important, and how upset my parents would be if I didn't drink it. He said he wouldn't tell my parents, and we agreed I would hand the empty carton back to him at the end of break for him to dispose of.

As time passed, Fortisips stopped being able to fulfil my dietary requirements, and before the end of primary school I was upgraded to Calshakes. These are made with 240ml of preferably full fat milk, (not that you'll be surprised by this, fat being something of a recurrent theme already in this book) into which is added a sachet of chocolate flavoured powder. The two are shaken together and the result is a slightly dissatisfying, ostensibly chocolate milkshake. They are a lot better tasting than Fortisip, and at 598.2 calories a pop (Fortisips are a mere 300) I'd go so far as to say they are probably the best tasting and most beneficial supplement. At first my parents gave me one every night before bed with my jumbo mars bar, but a week of vomiting onto my pillow from sheer volume led them to replace my milk at breakfast time instead. It has remained a morning, and now also mid-afternoon, (and when times are rough early evening) staple ever since.

Over time I have experienced a range of different types of supplement, from the reasonable in Calshake to the outright, probably against the Geneva convention, horrors of Calogen and Pro-cal shots. It's safe to say that fat content does not equate to tastiness - indeed the higher the amount of fat the worse the flavour seems to be. And let's not get started on texture. For some reason, smaller dose drinks (Calogen, with your PVA glue consistency, I'm looking at you) leave awful films coating the drinkers mouth, almost to mock a person for failing to digest enough fat through natural means. Sometimes, when I'm an inpatient, nurses ask if my supplements taste good. I always offer them a sample, but I've yet to have someone take me up on this. I think the smell is enough to suggest it's hardly gourmet, but it would be interesting to see medical staff give them a go.

Of course, for all my moaning, I do realise that taking these supplements is both important and much easier than the alternatives. Maintaining good weight is vital as fat is what helps a person have an immune system. Poor weight therefore equates to poor lung health, as the energy required to keep lung bugs at bay is hard to find. Some CF patients have nasogastric tubes which they use to deliver extra calories in the form of liquid feed, usually overnight, allowing the patient to keep up with their calories without having to worry about forcing too much extra food in. NG tubes are soft plastic tubes which are inserted up the nostril and down the throat into the stomach. I have twice tried to put one in, but despite my best efforts I couldn't get it down. In fairness, my nasal passageways suffer from scarring from three operations and a nasty break from a roller blading accident when I was 10. In the recovery room after my last sinus surgery, the ENT surgeon told me my nasal passageways were "an exciting mess" and that he had much enjoyed the challenge of operating on me. As compliments go it was odd, but I'll take it.

Failing an NG tube, the alternative is a PEG or a Button. These are direct tubes to the stomach through the abdomen. This allows for feed to be pumped straight in, again allowing extra calories to be consumed without the need to force yet more food in. I believe they are very effective, and a lot of CF patients have them. Indeed, the concept of having a button of my own has been floated a few times now. For no good reason, I'm reluctant to have a semi-permanent direct line in to my stomach, even though one does make sense. It feels a little bit more serious than necking the supplement drinks, but who knows what the future will hold. My dietitian believes it will take the effort out of eating, commenting that this can become a "chore". This is true, and I have to agree, but I find the concept of eating eventually becoming a chore slightly amusing. Every appointment since I can remember dietitians and doctors have asked me about my appetite. How is it? Is it good? I always reply it's fine, but to be honest I don't have a clue, having not been hungry since about 1996.

Generally, though, Primary school went well for me, and I was very happy. The only slight hiccup came when I was still in infants and my parents discovered that a girl in the year below me, called Sarah, also had CF. The chance of two unrelated children with CF attending the same school in an urban area with a huge number of primary schools is almost impossible, yet somehow it happened. I first discovered that Sarah also had CF when we were both invited to tea at our mutual friends' house. A set of sisters, close enough in age to be only a school year apart, we made a nice little foursome. Their mother had been good enough to do a little research into our shared condition and provided Sarah and I with huge portions of cheesy chips and burgers for tea, whilst her own daughters ate smaller, healthier meals with considerably less chips and a side salad. Sarah and I became firm friends, our mutual appreciation for Creon, understanding of physio and respect for how much time hospital appointments take forming a good foundation for a normal friendship. We played together in the playground every day, and I found great relief in learning I was not so unusual.

However, during the 1990s a greater understanding of the nature of CF bugs was being developed. Up until then CF was still considered more of a childhood illness as life expectancy was so low. As a result, camps were set up to allow CF sufferers the opportunity to get together and enjoy physical exercise, group physiotherapy sessions and generally get some relief from being with other young people who fully understood and could empathise with all the cruel effects of the condition. Although these camps were most popular in America, my parents were offered the chance to take me on one when I was still quite young. This sounds, on the face of it, like a wonderful idea. After all, who better to chat with and vent to than other young CF patients? This is not a unique concept. All other major illnesses – cancer, parkinsons, depression etc. have support groups for sufferers. No one can understand what a person is going through unless they themselves have walked in those shoes. Unfortunately for CF patients though, what was happening at these camps was simply a huge lung bug party. Patients were unknowingly swapping bacteria, sadly creating mutated, antibiotic resistant strains of already dangerous bugs. One bug, burkholderia cepacia, was tracked and shown to be more prevalent in patients who had attended CF camps than those who hadn't. Cepacia is a particularly nasty bug, and one of the three most likely to cause death in a patient. As a result of these findings cross infection measures began to be introduced into hospitals and people with CF were heavily discouraged from mixing. There was some disagreement over this, and there are some articles from even the early 2000s where doctors argue that actually the psychological toll of being separated out is worse than the physical danger of being together, but the huge leaps forward in medications over the last 15 years have now rendered these arguments entirely defunct. We no longer live in a time where very early death from CF is as prevalent, and therefore precautions are vital.

With this new research coming out, mine and Sarah's parents agreed that they didn't want to expose either of us to any risk, and unfortunately Sarah was withdrawn and moved to another primary school. Initially I was very angry that this had happened, despite my parents explaining that we would make each other poorly. I'd become accustomed to playing with her every day, and missed her, but I saw Sarah a few more times in clinic (in the distance, my parents were very firm and kept me away from the play table), and I could see that she was not looking too well. As young as I was, I could already see that there is a range of illness level within CF, even amongst children. I didn't want to cough like she did, and so abided by my parent's rule that we mustn't interact. Not long after she vanished from clinic, and I never saw her again.

This isolation is a unique feature of CF, and to me feels like one of the biggest hardships. Even for myself, a person who has been so well for so long, it is difficult to have no one who truly understands and will just listen without any explanations needed. Since Sarah I have never even spoken to a single other person with CF. Although the internet has helped a bit with this, there's nothing quite the same as a face to face chat. This is especially hard on CF patients who are that bit older, and remember being teenagers who sat and chatted in the communal rooms during their inpatient stays.

When CF patients go to hospital for appointments nowadays we are separated into different clinics based on what bugs we're growing, and then sit in separate clinic rooms. We arrive at staggered times to avoid standing near each other at the reception desk, and if we need more meds then there is often a nurse or health care assistant who goes to the hospital pharmacy for us. For hospital admissions, we are again separated out into different rooms with our own en-suite, and carriers of more obscure bugs (like me, for example) are not allowed to be admitted onto the CF ward (despite its separate rooms) at all and instead go elsewhere as an extra precaution. Back in the 1990s and early 2000s, before cross infection risks were fully understood, a much more blasé attitude was adopted. Clinic appointments at the children's unit included a lot of time in a communal waiting room, sitting together around a table with a play specialist enjoying blowing bubbles, modelling playdough and colouring whilst our parents chatted in seats round the edge of the room. We'd take it in turns to see the physio, the doctor and the dietitian and generally had a good afternoon all round.

My move to the adult clinic was quite a shock, with its separate rooms, clinics based specifically around different bugs and absolutely no contact with other patients. Obviously, this is much, much more sensible and things have now moved on to the extent that my CF team asks all CF patients to wear a surgical mask when walking around the hospital to further limit cross infection risks. It's really quite incredible to think how far understanding of cystic fibrosis has come on in just the last 20 years. What hasn't come on, unfortunately, is a more general appreciation of the condition by the NHS, particularly in relation to prescription charges.

When the NHS was first set up, there were certain conditions that were recognised as life-long illnesses that required regular medication for the entirety of a patient's life. These illnesses meant that the patient was granted free prescriptions for the whole of their lives. Diabetes, hypoparathyroidism and epilepsy are some of the more common. At the time, cystic fibrosis was thought of as just a childhood illness. No one, or at least almost no one, lived into adulthood with the condition, and so prescriptions were automatically free as they were being given to children. When the Cystic Fibrosis Trust was first set up, back in 1964, one of its first remits was to campaign for free prescriptions for adults, as the founders of the charity were certain that one day CF would be an illness survived by many into adulthood. We're now 55 years on, and most patients not only reach adulthood, but many can live way beyond even the wildest dreams of the initial trustees. Despite this, we are still not given free prescriptions. Fortunately, pre-paid certificates are available allowing a one-off sum to be paid every 12 months. At £115 it's not a mind-blowing sum of money, and I do appreciate that it is only a tiny fraction of the amount that my drugs actually cost, but it still irks me every year when I renew. What was awful, however, was my first adult experience of collecting a prescription.

I am an August birthday, and so turned 18 just before heading off down the country to start university. My first act during fresher's week was to join a GP Surgery and put in a prescription. I blithely turned up at the pharmacy three days later to collect my nine item prescription, and was shocked to be asked to hand over £71 for my drugs. Taken aback I tried to argue my way out of paying, but no, it was money or no meds. I paid, thankful that my student loan had actually come in, and walked back to my halls lugging my huge box of meds and panicking about how I could possibly afford to keep paying this every month. Fortunately, a quick internet search allowed me to set myself up with a prepaid certificate, and I was eventually able to claim the money back, but for a few hours I was certain that my CF was going to bankrupt me.

Sarah's departure from primary school had a ripple effect on my life in that our little foursome was broken up. The younger sister blamed me, and we parted ways. I stuck up for myself though, explaining that CF is complicated and I wasn't allowed to meet anyone with CF anymore, because we'll just make each other poorly. I did stay friends with the older sister, but we were never quite the same, and although we went on to the same secondary school we moved into different circles.

By secondary school I was well versed in the need to speak up about my CF, and defend things that seemed unreasonable (or disgusting) to my peers. My primary school had been supportive, and my friends appreciated my condition, but as we got older they were already starting to make odd comments about it, and I was starting to feel a little got at. At the start of my second week at secondary school, an older boy (a lofty year 8!) sought me out to pick on me about my cough. He had previously had a to-do with my older brother, and came to me in order to continue the feud. This was a hard experience for me, having been sheltered so well at primary school, but in fairness was a harder experience for him. "Eww! Gross! Stop coughing you'll spread your manky disease," he mocked by the lockers. I was shocked at his meanness, and livid that he was choosing to pick on my CF. I pulled myself up to my full height and spat "It's genetic" at him. As come backs go, it was weak. But the fist that I threw into his face at the same time made up for that. He retreated, and the story that the skinny year 7 girl with the cough was crazy and dangerous spread like wildfire, backed up by his remarkably long lasting black eye. After that incident, I was never bullied again. Fortunately, my teachers turned a blind eye to this episode, which at the time I thought was just really lucky, although in hindsight I'm sure they must have been aware of what had happened. I've never let anyone be mean to me about my CF since, and hopefully he has learnt not to be nasty to people who cough. Or perhaps he just learnt not to mess with skinny blondes. Either way, it was a valuable life lesson for both of us.

Despite the rocky start, I settled in well to the new school, throwing myself into both academic and extra-curricular activities alike, taking everything I did extremely seriously. My school had a reputation for very high academic standards, but sports were not up there for them. P.E was considered one of life's evils, and not really a subject. As a result, the whole school, teachers included, spent the annual sports day just sat on the field in the sun, enjoying a relaxed morning, paying only lip service to the track and field events going on round them.

My fellow classmates embraced this attitude wholeheartedly. All the girls were lovely, and academically they were brilliant, but not one had a competitive bone in their body when it came to sports. As a result, we always came dead last as a team. By contrast, I am a horribly competitive person – I can't even bare to lose at Connect Four to a child- and in year 9 I decided to remedy the situation. From year 9 form roles were introduced, and I set my sights on becoming form sports captain, determined to remedy our embarrassing past defeats, carefully planning a campaign to muster support. This I put into full swing, lobbying for votes from every other member of my form, despite there being no one else even remotely interested in running against me. Unsurprisingly a land slide victory got me the job. With sports day on the horizon, I cajoled, bribed and generally harassed the girls in my form over a number of weeks to sign up for events and got our team ready.

On the day itself, however, my team decided that the warmth of the sun and comfort of the playing field were far too good to be left, and not a single one attended their event. I ran around like a headless chicken, pleading with them to mobilise themselves, clipboard in hand, but my pleas fell on deaf ears. I went off to see what I could do, and discovered that the teachers had also decided they would enjoy the sun, entrusting the actual running of the events to members of the upper sixth, presumably with the promise that they wouldn't have to undertake any exercise themselves. The sixth formers all had lists of the entrants for every event, but to my delight they had no idea who anyone was. I began at the opposite end of the playground, and throughout the course of the morning took part in every single event, using an assumed name for each. The final event was the only one I had actually entered in to – the 800m. This took place on the main field in full view of all the teachers. I lined up at the start line, already knackered, and set off at full speed with the gun. By 400m, I was falling behind, the effort of running, jumping, throwing and skipping all morning catching up with me. I could see some of my teachers starting to stand up and watch me. I finished, a good few minutes behind everyone else, and was startled to see the teachers all stood up to clap me. My physics teacher came over and put his arm round my shoulder, leading me off from the track. "Well done, Abi, I know that must have been really hard for you," he said, offering me a drink of water and a chair. Embarrassed by the attention, I didn't really know what to say, thinking I hadn't done that bad a job all things considering. I grimaced and excused myself, and the teachers all watched me limp back to the company of my form.

The next day, results all in, we had our year group assembly. My form had come second overall, which considering we'd had only one athlete wasn't too bad. The head of year gave out the certificate for the winning form, then produced another one from his lectern. "We also have a certificate for exceptional effort," he proclaimed, "Please can Abi come up to the front". Confused I headed up to stand next to him. He was smiling at me, and he had in his hand a certificate for running 800m. I looked at him nonplussed, my 800m clearly having been nothing worth celebrating. He shook my hand as he handed it to me and quietly whispered he and the rest of the staff appreciated how difficult running so far must have been with my poorly lungs. Mortified, I thanked him and headed back to my shamelessly grinning, cheering classmates, wondering what the collective noun for benefits cheats was.

Throughout my life I have often come across people who understand what CF is, but don't appreciate that it has a wildly different effect on every patient. As such I am often recipient of unnecessary, but very well meaning, acts of kindness. As an adult, I once entered a raffle at my local pharmacy. I wasn't terribly interested in the prizes, but as a very regular user of the service I felt I ought to show some support. A week later I received a phone call from the pharmacist. She wanted to check I would bring my car to collect my latest prescription, as I had also won a large amount from the raffle. I was slightly surprised, but turned up the next day to collect everything. To my disbelief, the pharmacy team congratulated me on winning all three of the top prizes, three lovely hampers of chocolates, smellies and even a very cosy dressing gown. I didn't know what to say, as I knew this wasn't possible. "Are you sure?" I ventured, "this seems extremely unlikely." The head pharmacist flapped at me, assuring me that I had definitely won all three. I tried to disagree, but she took on a firm look. "Some people just need a bit of luck in their lives Mrs Halstead, and obviously this is your time." I could see her mind was made up, and so thanked them all profusely, and they helped me load my car with medication and goodies. I drove off, guiltily putting my single raffle ticket in the bin when I got home.

Despite the sports day fiasco of year 9, my teachers did a good job of letting my live a normal life at school. They didn't make a fuss over me, to the point where I ended up carrying a team mates bag as well as my own on our Duke of Edinburgh award, as the girl had asthma and couldn't possibly complete the hike and carry her bag. I was willing to do this for her as I just wanted the endless bickering about exactly what our coordinates were to be over, and to sit down at a nice (ha!) campsite. But as we walked I did slightly roll my eyes at the CF girl carrying a double load even though our accompanying teacher only had a compass and a spare jumper.

This illusion that I was considered to be just another normal pupil was shattered though at the end of year awards evening in my AS Level year. Every year all the highest achieving, hardest working etc. pupils from each year were given a certificate in front of all the parents. It was a real honour to be invited, and being a mega geek I attended it every year. In year 12 I attended as usual and was taken aback to be singled out for a very special award for "personal endeavour" as I had overcome "great personal challenges" during my time at school. Embarrassed I turned scarlet and walked nervously out onto stage, rudely forgetting to thank the distinguished guest who was handing out all the certificates. The shield I received, engraved "Abilail", was a very kind thought by well-meaning teachers, but to me it felt like I had been secretly singled out as "different", and therefore "weird". Looking back with adult eyes I can see that of course I was singled out. Every teacher would have known who I was, it would have been foolish for the school not to have made all the staff aware of the girl with a serious disease roaming the school, missing lessons for hospital appointments and potentially vanishing for weeks or months at a time. (This, fortunately, never happened, but most CF patients miss vast amounts of school as they get older and iller.) In hindsight, although I thought my school was just a wonderful, friendly place, the fact that almost every teacher would nod at me or say, "Hello Abi," when I walked past, whether or not I'd ever been taught by them, should have been a clue that I was not considered to be just another normal pupil. The shield sits on a shelf in my old bedroom at my parents' house, next to my Judo trophy, a strange and slightly unsettling reminder that despite my best efforts, I'm not the same as everyone else, and I never ever will be.

-3-

JOHN

At the age of 15 I met my first proper boyfriend, the man I went on to marry. Our initial meeting was a chance one at a church event in Sheffield. We both got into the back of the same car on the way to an activity, simply because I didn't know anyone else there, and he had a mammoth crush on the girl driving, and was trying to worm his way in with her. We hit it off immediately, and the long traffic jam we got stuck in, causing a 15 minute journey to become a 45 minute one, seems like fate. We chatted for the whole time, oblivious to the driver and her other passenger. We didn't speak again for the rest of the event, but I saw him watching me during the buffet tea, observing me taking my Creon in a curious but not disturbed way. Just as I was about to leave he nipped over and we swapped numbers.

I was only young, and was initially flattered that a lad some whole three-and-a-half years older than me even wanted to know my name, let alone actually be interested in going out with me. Plus he had a car, so what wasn't to love? On the negative side though he lived in Spalding, which is a good three hours away from Manchester. My parents were willing to fork out for the train fare though, and John was happy to drive up and down the country to see me.

At first we just texted casually, but then my parents got broadband, and we started spending evening after evening on MSN. My brothers moaned I was hogging the computer, but I swore blind that I needed it for my homework, despite the obvious constant pinging of messages. Early on John asked me about my future career plans, and I took the opportunity to tell him about my hopes of university, caveating it heavily with the phrase "if my health allows." He took the bait and we stopped dodging around the elephant in the room. Of course, "if my health allows" was a greatly exaggerated phrase. I was fit, healthy and well, and my cystic fibrosis was still just something I took a lot of pills for, ate tonnes and did lots of physiotherapy and exercise because of, but it was not actually affecting my life in a particularly tangible way. Although of course it was possible that the pendulum could swing back at any second, it seemed highly unlikely that I wouldn't be able to go to university because of it. However, I knew that the time when illness takes over would eventually come, and was unwilling to commit time to a long-distance relationship if the lad was going to be scared off by the mere concept of future health problems. Surprisingly he wasn't, and we had a very frank discussion about what cystic fibrosis is, and what it means in reality. Impressed by his determination to continue "courting" me, despite the fact that I had broken all social etiquette and discussed GI tracts, mucus and life expectancy with him, I agreed to meet up with him at another church event, this time in Llandudno, and we officially started "going out".

Although I started strong with explanations about my health, our conversations were all very hypothetical, and I balked at the thought of actually talking about things like poo. It was still early days, and there are limits. John is actually a plumber, although at the time was still an apprentice, so he was unlikely to be too grossed out by all things faecal, but I was still keen to preserve some level of romantic dignity.

I may not have mentioned it out loud, but inside I was suffering from almost stomach ulcer inducing levels of anxiety about the subject. Living so far apart meant that when we did meet up, we spent the whole weekend together at each other's houses. This was nice, but did mean that I couldn't avoid the issue for long, and soon found myself in his house, needing to poo. Now pooing, for someone with cystic fibrosis, can be quite an unpleasant experience. We are unable to properly digest our food, which results in, amongst other things, a high likelihood of either diarrhoea, extreme constipation or sometimes both. Even "normal" bowel movements are smellier than average, as there is a higher amount of undigested food and fat left in the stool. As well as this (as if this wasn't embarrassing enough in a fledgling relationship) the need to keep up with our vast calorie intake requires huge amounts of food to be consumed, and so people with CF go to the toilet a lot more regularly, sometimes with an extreme sense of urgency, if you catch my drift. In order to avoid too much embarrassment too early on I got into the habit of eating less on weekends when I saw him, and started setting my alarm for 3 o'clock in the morning so I could use the toilet without fear of judgement. This worked at first, but after too many trips where I bumped into his father on the landing in the middle of the night, I realised he was just going to have to take me as I am and abandoned my late-night excursions.

As time went on we realised that we were very well suited, and deeply in love. After a few years John started talking about taking the next step and tying the knot. In theory this sounded fantastic, but I was reluctant. I knew what the future holds, and was worried that he hadn't grasped just how horrible it will undoubtedly be. I had been extremely well for the whole of our relationship, indeed he hadn't even attended a hospital appointment with me – my hospital appointments are on weekdays, and at the time were over 100 miles away from his place of work. The only real insight into the potential effect of my condition that he had had was witnessing me have a small emotional breakdown over a new bug I started to grow. It was called burkholderia gladioli, and not only could my doctor not seem to get rid of it, he seemed unwilling to give me much information about it, instead telling me not to worry. This was an ongoing problem throughout my time at the child clinic. My consultant was a kind man, gentle mannered, softly spoken and hardworking. He clearly preferred younger children though – the colour he turned when asking me, now I was a young woman with a boyfriend, if I'd thought about contraception was incredible, and not long after I started seeing a female doctor whenever he had one working in the clinic. When I finally moved up to the adult clinic at the age of 18 I bought him a box of chocolates and wrote him a nice thankyou card. He took them and squeezed my hand, reminiscing that it had been a long time since I had sat on his knee during clinic appointments (apparently quite an unusual thing for a child in a hospital to do) and telling me, uncharacteristically sternly, to stay sensible and keep looking after myself as well as I always have. He then wished me all the best for the future in a slightly nasally voice and headed off up to the children's ward.

Perhaps as a result of his kindly nature, he appeared to be almost phobic of telling children he'd known their whole lives the full truth about their illness. Or at least, he was never too honest with his answers to any of my more difficult questions, preferring instead to stall and talk about something else. To combat this absence of information, I relied on the internet to fill the void. Unfortunately, burkholderia gladioli is something of a rare bug, and I struggled to find much more than passing references, no matter how much I trawled through medical journals. As a result, I became paranoid that it was going to kill me, and convinced myself that my doctor had decided that it would be kinder not to let me know how quickly this was going to happen. In reality, my doctor could see that this new bug hadn't touched my lung function, and rather than subject me to eradication treatment for something that appeared to be merely chilling out in my respiratory system, he set about working hard to try and pinpoint where I'd caught it from, never having had a patient with it before. He asked me to have my boyfriend sort himself out with a cough swab to see if he was somehow the carrier of it. John willingly did this, and was exposed to how difficult it can be to get some GPs to do obscure tests without a strongly worded letter from a consultant, but he didn't grow it and its origins remain a mystery.

Other than this brief meltdown – I was only just 16, but even at the height of melodramatic teenage angst I realised after a few months that nothing had changed, I was not dying, and just got on with life as I always have done. (13 years on I still have my little burkholderia hitch-hiker. It sometimes flares up a bit, and needs stamping down on with IVs, but generally it's pretty content to just hang out in my lungs without causing too much trouble.) However, apart from this high tension few months, during which John spent quite a lot of time sitting and holding me as I alternated between crying and quietly raging at how unfair the hand life has dealt me was, I didn't have any real problems. I was concerned that he thought I would forever continue to coast through life as easily as I have done so far, not realising that I will one day need to spend a lot of time in hospital, become dependent on bottled oxygen and eventually die young from my disease.

After yet another phone conversation at university with John telling me it made sense for us to just jump in and get married, I went into the communal kitchen to make a brew and clear my head. My friend from further down the corridor joined me, and sensing a problem, asked what was wrong. We sat together at the kitchen table and I poured out all of my fears and worries, my dilemma at wanting to get married but not wanting to lumber John with my illness in the future, what about children? Is it ok to get married to someone knowing you're going to die young, would it not be fairer to let him meet someone else…? The list kept going, and I had tears in my eyes. I looked up from my tea to see her sitting, open mouthed, clearly unable to process everything I was saying. We were both young in our year group, still a way off 19, and were not that close. As it was only early February we'd actually only known each other less than 5 months. To my shock she started to sob, and I realised I'd never really talked to anyone at university about the grim details of my condition, only giving the glossy top line. Unlike me, she wasn't really emotionally prepared for a late-night conversation about marriage, medicine and mortality. Fortunately, another flatmate came in. He's the most relaxed lad I've ever met, but at that moment was awkwardly walking, or more correctly, waddling sideways, carrying an array of dirty cups and plates from his room, looking extremely sheepish. He spotted the tears and paused, clearly unsure what the best course of action was. We all looked at each other, and after a moment's silence I asked him why he wasn't walking properly. He informed me that his belt had broken earlier in the day, he hadn't got around to changing it, but actually he realised his trousers wouldn't stay up without it. He therefore had to waddle with his legs open wide to avoid embarrassment as his hands were too full to hold them up. He told this bizarre tale in such a matter of fact way that I couldn't help but laugh. The tension was lifted and he joined in our cup of tea, and then offered us something a bit stronger. We never talked about my outburst again. John proposed at the end of the Spring term, which I happily accepted, and we got married in the summer of 2010, at the tender ages of 19 and 23. I realised in that evening that actually, I am in love, life is too short to say no, and that yes, my life is perhaps a little bit more complicated than my peers, but that John seems to be happy with that, and can handle a lot more than I'd given him credit for.

Although I've not had any reactions quite as extreme as that since, life with CF is often lonely, even when healthy and surrounded by friends. I rarely talk about medical or health related things with my friends after the initial explanations, but when necessity forces things out almost every sentence begins with "It's nothing to worry about, but...", or "Don't worry, this is actually really normal, but..." And, it's true, all of my CF treatment is "normal" (or at least normal within a given value), but I still sometimes want someone to tell me it's ok and that they appreciate how frustrated or occasionally how scared I am. That they recognise that keeping healthy enough to live an ordinary life requires a lot of work, but that it is "normal" to have to do this, rather than me having to both explain and reassure in the same breath.

I may not talk too much about my health, but the underlying knowledge that I have a major health condition regularly causes friends and acquaintances to share their health problems, hospital trips and antibiotic courses with me, often in great detail. I'm always sympathetic, but I try not to offer anything too much about my own situation in return. CF is so all encompassing that even someone as well as myself has had a diverse range of medical experiences, and any comparisons can quickly descend into a bizarre game of illness top trumps. This is especially true when a friend tells me they're having to undergo two weeks of an oral antibiotic such as flucloxacillin. They will usually give me a run-down of all their side effects, proudly telling me that they know how I feel now to be taking antibiotics, and openly wondering how I do it all the time as they don't know how they could do it. It always feels like it would be churlish to take away from their experience by telling them I've been on double their dose for over 20 years, and side effects just become normal, so I tend to just smile and nod.

Long-term antibiotic use is a confusing situation for the uninitiated. We are bombarded in the news so regularly with stories about how bad antibiotics are, how over prescribed they are and how they are therefore becoming less and less effective. Obviously this is all true, however there are some caveats to this statement, and the long term use of antibiotics in patients with chronic illness like CF is one of them. We are constantly at risk of infections, and are almost always actually fighting them in our lungs. I've had the same bug sitting in my lungs for 13 years now, and every day my immune system is waging a small war against it and any sneaky extra bugs, aided and abetted by the antibiotics I take. Because of this risk and situation CF patients take a lot of antibiotics. I inhale antibiotics twice a day, alternating between two different ones on a monthly basis, and until recently took a catch-all oral antibiotic twice a day as well. In addition to this I take another oral antibiotic three times a week to help supress the inflammation in my lungs, and whenever I start to feel unwell I immediately start taking another oral antibiotic or two.

When I feel unwell this can either be the sign of a new infection, or of my existing infections getting stronger and gaining a bit of ground (this is called an exacerbation). I have yet more pumped into me intravenously whenever I'm actually "ill", although I prefer to think of it as when I'm a bit under the weather. Describing myself as "ill", when there are so many people with CF who are really, *really* ill feels melodramatic. But yes, there is a real problem with infections becoming antibiotic resistant. This is frightening for everybody, but particularly for those of us who are more susceptible to infections. Although part of the blame can lie with the over prescription of antibiotics, a lot of blame also lies with people not completing their course. This is a huge danger to everyone as it allows bugs to mutate, making them less susceptible to antibiotics. So please, if you are prescribed antibiotics, take them properly and finish your course, even if you feel better. If you don't, or ever haven't, then please give yourself a slap from me.

Although John was wonderfully supportive from the beginning, he has, over time, adopted a rather blasé attitude to hospital visits. So much so that even minor operations don't rank high enough on our list of important life events for him to stick around during them. When I had my gall bladder out he drove me to the hospital, pulled into the drop off bay, gave me a quick peck on the cheek and told me to call him when I was done. After the surgery, I was wheeled back to the ward and woozily asked the visitor sat at the bed opposite me (who was lovingly clasping his partner's hand as she waited to be taken up for whatever minor day case elective surgery she was waiting for) to reach into my bag and pass me my phone. He raced over and willingly passed it to me, and I thanked him, casually mentioning that I needed to phone my husband to let him know the procedure had gone well, and I was now sans gall bladder. The man looked disgustedly at me, wanting to know why my husband wasn't at my side. I shrugged and said he was too busy for minor things like gall bladders, and the man inhaled sharply and shook his head, before walking back across to his also horrified looking partner. I made my brief phone call, acutely aware of the sympathetic smiles and headshakes the patients and family members in the four other occupied beds were giving me. When John arrived in the middle of the afternoon to sit with me whilst I was discharged and then take me to my normal CF hospital for post-operative care, the other patients all eyed him coldly and the bay took on a distinctly frosty feel. "What have I done?" he whispered to me. "Nothing, noone's looking at you," I lied guiltily, "they're just stressed." I briefly made eye contact with the phone man opposite, who was leaving with his newly discharged wife, shaking his head at John as he left. In fairness, although I bounce back quickly from general anaesthetics, I spend the first few hours looking hideously ill. I'm always as white as a sheet, lips the same colour as my face, which blends in perfectly with the pillowcase behind it. I'm woozy, my blood pressure is always very low (blood pressure is often lower in CF patients, normally as a result of salt mismana-gement) and this time the nurses had given me oxygen for a few hours to help. All in all, I looked rough. But by that night I was absolutely fine, and quite frankly life is just too short, too busy, and hospital visits too frequent, for both of us just to drop everything and hang out there whenever something happens.

Less than a year later, when having nasal polyps removed again, the mother of the woman in the bed next to me took such pity on me being alone that she decided to adopt me for the day. Nasal polyps and sinus issues run hand and hand with CF because the sinuses and nasal passages are lined with epithelial cells, thus causing chronic sinusitis and the formation of vast numbers of polyps. To date I've had my sinuses scraped and the polyps removed three times, and I'm sure I will need them doing again in the future. The woman's own daughter was having a very minor procedure, and her surgery was later in the day than mine. The older woman was clearly very stressed by the whole experience, and sat by my bed for the whole time that her daughter was in theatre, stroking my head and giving me sips of water. I was actually fine, and really quite wanted to move about, despite being white as a sheet and rather bloody, but she seemed to need to occupy herself so I just lay still and listened to her as she told me her whole life story, her daughter's life story, and all about her two dogs.

Every time I did try to escape from the bed she gently pressed me down again and made soft soothing noises. Her daughter was returned to the ward and discharged only two hours later, slightly rolling her eyes at how much her mother was flapping over me, and the woman took pains to tuck me in tightly, fluff my pillow and make sure I was comfortable before she left. I smiled and thanked her, then waited until she had definitely left the building before getting out of bed and having a much-needed stretch, feeling rather fraudulent and avoiding eye contact with the other, slightly incredulous looking, patients in the bay as I did.

In fairness, I'm often told I look quite young for my age and the lady probably thought I needed a bit of mothering. At 28 I'm still getting ID'd for alcohol, which is a little embarrassing. Unless of course I'm buying it when I have the children with me, when the checkout assistant tends to look at the multitude of toddlers I've squashed into the four-seater trolley (these actually exist and are amazing) and practically cracks it open right there for me.

The longer we've been together, the more normal absolutely everything CF related has become for John. He gets involved in my treatments, and my life with CF has become ours. He rarely comes with me to clinic, but I go over everything that is said every time with him that night. He sometimes collects my prescription, often makes my Calshakes, harasses me daily to eat more and, when I'm doing home IVs, he will often take over pushing them in last thing at night when I'm feeling too tired.

In recent months, I have had my scariest experience with CF to date, and it's caused both of us to take a pause and refocus. Late one night we got into bed chatting casually about our days, when John commented that I'd seemed very well recently. Since having the children my health has not been at its best. A combination of two very close pregnancies, exhaustion, gall bladder troubles, sinus problems and huge weight loss have caused a few chest exacerbations (or increased infection levels), and for the first time in my life I have not paid quite such close daily attention to my medication, physio, exercise and weight management that cystic fibrosis requires. This has caused me to feel slightly unwell for quite some time, but John was right, in the past few weeks I'd felt better than I had for nearly three years. I smiled at him and agreed, lying down and snuggling into him as I did. In hind sight this was the perfect horror movie cliché, the girl pronouncing herself safe at last, just before the monster chops her head off and everyone jumps. I closed my eyes for sleep, then heard a strange gurgling sound, which seemed to emanate from deep inside my chest, and felt a sudden urge to cough. When I did, my hand filled with liquid, and I sat bolt upright, John switching on the light. My palm was filled with scarlet blood, and I was coughing more and more out. John froze, horrified at the sight of his wife apparently pouring blood from her lungs, then grabbed me a handful of tissues. I continued to cough blood into tissue after tissue for a good few minutes before the flow subsided. Unsure what to do, I phoned my CF centre and was put through to the doctor on call. The doctor reassured me that this was normal for a person with CF, and that I wasn't dying. I mentally disagreed with her assertion that this could be classed as "normal" for anyone, but her calmness soothed me. She set about establishing just how much blood had been lost, then, satisfied it wasn't significant enough that I was in any danger, she rang off to speak to the on-call consultant, promising to phone me back shortly.

Coughing up blood, or haemoptysis, is actually, as the doctor assured me, a very normal situation in cystic fibrosis. Infection in the lungs can cause the walls to become inflamed, and if the infection localises in a small area, the blood vessels in that area can be put under too much strain and pop, causing blood to flow into the lungs. This sounds terrible, but actually the amount of blood that comes from these vessels is usually very small (however large it may appear in the moment), and the infection that has caused the problem is normally treatable. Although I don't have much experience of this I had read about it before, but it actually happening was much more frightening and shocking than I had appreciated it could be. Approximately half of adults with CF routinely cough up blood streaked mucus as a result of minor haemoptysis. In odd cases, the amount of blood can be more than a cup. This is a "massive haemoptysis" and requires the patient to be hospitalised and a procedure called an embolization is performed to block off the vessel. My small experience was nothing to worry about, my consultant thinks I was just unlucky, and I was started on oral antibiotics for the infection and tranexamic acid to help stop any clots from breaking down, thus stopping any further bleeding.

At an appointment a month or so later, the consultant gave me a run-down of all the results from my hastily booked annual review tests. As an off-the-cuff comment in regard to my recent haemoptysis he enquired if I'd had any night sweats, as this is a sign of infection. I said a categorical no, but actually I had spent over a week after the haemoptysis waking up in the early hours, drenched in sweat. At the time, I put it down to stress brought on by the experience, and ignored it. Even as I was saying no I knew this was a stupid thing to do; I'd never lied to a doctor before in my life. But for some reason I couldn't bring myself to admit that I'd had a problem, or might actually have been ill. In fairness, the doctor had already arranged for me to come in for two weeks IVs, to start as soon as they had space and I'd managed to organise childcare, so I mentally told myself there was no need to go back over the past (even though it was actually quite recent). The oral antibiotics seemed to have cleared up the infection, or at least I'd stopped waking up sweating, and any residual infection would hopefully be cleared up by my new lot of oral antibiotics and the imminent IVs. It wasn't that bad anyway, I told myself on the way home, so what would be the point?

When I got home from the appointment, John could tell there was something not quite right. He asked about what the doctor had said, what all my results were. I told him everything that had been said, vaguely mentioning the doctor had mentioned night sweats. John immediately remembered that I had woken up for over a week sweaty in the night. I hadn't realised it had been so bad, but apparently I had moaned about it every morning, complaining I was shattered as a result. He wanted to know what the doctor had said to do if they happened in the future. I was a little stumped and had to admit I'd neglected to share that I'd been having them. Instantly, John got cross with me. Why didn't I tell the doctor? Why lie? What else have I been keeping secret? In response, I retorted angrily that he didn't understand and he needed to leave me alone.

We rowed about it for the rest of the evening. Since the children our rows have become less big blow outs and more small, cruel snipes as we joust in between entertaining the children, wiping their bottoms, walking the dog, prepping dinner, cleaning up, sorting laundry, calling customers to confirm plumbing work and wrangling our reluctant offspring through bath time and bed. I went to bed early to avoid talking about it, and could hear John stomping round in the kitchen, clearly still angry with me. He eventually joined me upstairs and curled round me under the covers. Eventually I couldn't ignore him any longer and stopped feigning sleep. It's ok, he said, just tell the doctor if it ever happens again. He understood that the new regime of coming into hospital every few months was weighing heavily on me, and I didn't want to think about things. But he also reminded me that he does understand. He is intrinsically linked to my health, and so are our children. I'm 28, and now is not the time to start messing about. Instead we need to dig deeper and work a bit harder, making peace with the new status quo, something we both know I haven't been doing.

-4-

THE WORLD OF WORK

Having completed my university degree I went out, portfolio in hand, into the design studios of London. The way into packaging and branding design, usually, is through a university degree, followed by internships at various design studios. The idea is that the young designer will eventually fall lucky and be at a studio they are suited to at the time when the studio is in need of a new junior. I happily spent the summer traipsing around the city, touting my portfolio at interview after interview, and lined myself up with a solid 6 months of 2 to 4 week internship slots. I got on well enough, enjoying the different experiences that studios offered and generally got wrapped up in my new, exciting life. As I was already married, and John's job was not in London, we set up home out in the countryside and I joined the daily commuting grind with a skip in my step, feeling like a real adult. But as time went on, I became a little worried. My internships were not leading to jobs, and I was having to do more interviews to fill my time after the current ones ended. I interviewed again and again, filling a whole year with slots. I was confused. I hadn't left university expecting to walk straight into a job, but I knew I was good enough for a job, and had gathered more than enough experience to be worthy of one. Even more confusingly, studios I'd already interned at kept in touch with me and offered me chances to come back and work for them again whenever I was free. Most worryingly, studios began to give me gifts when I left them. These started out small, the odd box of chocolates, but soon moved on to expensive bottles of alcohol (not just freebies from their clients) and even some Apple technology.

I met up with some of my university friends about 10 months after graduating for a post work drink, carrying my snazzy new bit of gifted design kit. My friends, now employed, admired it, commenting that the most they'd ever got was a card and the occasional nice pen. Surprised, I reeled off the long list of gifts I had been the recipient of. My friends were taken aback, especially when I revealed that my portfolio had doubled in size, filling with work I had done on placements – all signed off with permission from design directors to use as I pleased. Again, my friends were a bit surprised I was not only working on my own ideas on placements, but also allowed to take them with me. It's no secret that interns sneakily take projects they've had even a tiny stake in to showcase in their portfolio, but it's not really allowed and interviewers can be a bit funny about it. I, on the other hand, was actually being encouraged to do this, and at one point at the end of an internship the design director took my hard drive from my bag and downloaded not only two projects, but every single font and image I might ever want from the system. He handed it back to me with a conspiratorial wink and a quiet ssh! This was actually stealing, but as technically I wasn't the thief my conscience was clean and I kept it quiet.

On the train home I thought about this disconcerting situation, and the penny finally dropped with a bang. Were the people employing me as an intern being frightened off by my CF? Branding designers are, by their very nature, inquisitive people who spend large amounts of time researching into the companies and products they are designing for in order to tease out exactly what message their client's designs should be giving. Most projects start with heavy research before any of the many initial design routes make it to paper. Within a few days of every placement the designers around me would mention my cough. After I'd explained it was my CF, there would usually be a few basic questions, and then we'd all get back to work. I suspect that what was happening was that the designers were then googling cystic fibrosis to within an inch of its life. And there I was, sat in the middle of people who were most likely learning every grim detail of my condition, it's inevitable ending, and most importantly, the huge amounts of time a "normal" CF patient spends sitting in a hospital having IVs. In the five years I worked as a packaging designer I was only once asked to explain CF to more than a basic level, yet every internship and eventually freelance job I left the designers would almost all hug me and tell me to look after my chest, and take it easy, and whenever I was at a studio during an employee's birthday I was always cut a double portion of cake. The regularity of these occurrences seems more than coincidental.

A few days after I came to this realisation I went back to a studio I'd spent a bit of time at and sat down with a design director I'd got on quite well with. Without making eye contact, he coughed and confirmed that there might be a slight, non-work related, issue with hiring me, although he wouldn't be specific what it was, and swore he would deny ever having said that if I brought it up publicly. The London design world is a small one, and designers like a bit of a gossip. His advice was to take advantage of that by asking for more money on placements in the future, and he hoped something would come up. That night I went home and repackaged myself as a freelance junior designer. This is not a job that actually exists, but a lot of the studios I'd interned at were happy to take me on anyway. I'm under no illusion that at first this was out of sympathy, but as time passed I got more confident, upped my rates and worked at a lot of different studios. I had a fantastic working experience, made a lot of friends, and enjoyed working on a lot of exciting projects, perhaps more than I would have done if I'd stayed in the same studio for years, not months or weeks, at a time.

The difficulty I had in securing a full-time job is not unique to me. I understand a lot of other people with CF and other chronic illnesses struggle to find full time employment. The necessity of hospital appointments and stays means we need to take a lot more time off than most. We don't know when we will next be ill, or when we will need to drop our lives to deal with a new health problem. In addition, the effects of conditions like CF aren't fully understood by most normal people. It's difficult to go to an interview for a job and then have to explain you will need time off when the interviewer doesn't understand why that would be. And let's be honest, job interviews are just not the time to talk about poo and mucus. I understand why this is difficult for employers, but it does mean those with chronic conditions are left feeling more helpless, and more isolated.

The only downside of my freelance life was the constant pressure of changing jobs every few weeks. I actually enjoyed the experience as I love getting to know people, but it was still tiring. It's the nature of the beast, as freelancers are always joining teams who are already over stretched. The need to always be at your best is mentally exhausting, especially when you've made your job up in the first place. This, combined with my car, train, and either tube or walk (the walk to the train at the end was usually a sprint) from out in the country to central London, began to leave me feeling more than a little run down. I was up early and back late every day, soon perfecting the art of sleeping on the train. I would get up, shower and dress in a daze, drive to the station and be asleep on the train before it had even left the platform. The other commuters probably didn't notice, being entrenched in similar routines themselves, but I did once wake up to a very smartly dressed man in an expensive suit politely tapping me to tell me we'd reached the end of the line in London. Embarrassingly, I was actually asleep on his shoulder. I had no recollection of him even getting on the train, and could only apologise and hope I hadn't dribbled. He didn't seem to mind, although he probably wondered what I was doing on the early train as I was wearing my designer's uniform of ripped jeans and a hoodie in amongst a sea of black suits. The only time I did get funny looks from fellow passengers was when I attempted to streamline my morning routine by taking my nebuliser on the train.

Modern nebulisers are small, portable devices that allow a person to inhale medication. The medication (in this case an antibiotic called tobramycin) usually comes as a liquid in a small plastic cartridge which is broken and poured into the nebuliser's chamber. Just like a deodorant aerosol can, the liquid is then fired through a metal piece (the aerosol) which forces the liquid into tiny molecules giving it the appearance of cold steam. It then travels a little further down a tube and out through a mouthpiece where the patient inhales the vapour. If the medication is an antibiotic, as it was in this case, a filter is used to stop any of the antibiotic escaping and being inhaled by other people. When I was first given my nebuliser, it added 15 minutes to my morning routine (and took another 15 minutes of my evening), and I thought taking it on the train would be the perfect way to avoid sacrificing precious sleep time. I sat on the train, pulled down the normally useless table from the chair in front of me, set up my nebuliser and began to take my antibiotic. The man I was sat next to moved. This was an unexpected positive to me, extra space always being a bonus, but when the person in front also moved I started to feel a little judged. The commuters across the aisle stared openly, and the blokes behind also moved. Too late, I realised John was right to be dubious about the idea. I brazened it out, finishing my neb and enjoying the ability to spread out a little. When I got to the studio I washed the nebuliser parts in the sink. This in itself got odd looks from the other kitchen users, and I gave the whole idea up as a dud.

I'm now quite a few years on from my first experiences of nebulised antibiotics. Nowadays I alternate monthly between a different nebulised antibiotic and a podhaler, both of which I inhale twice daily. My new antibiotic comes as a powder, requiring me to mix it up with sodium chloride solution before I nebulise it. This is a bit of a faff as the solution must be transferred to the powder bottle by means of a needle and syringe, which adds time to the treatment. The whole thing, washing up after included, takes about 15-20 minutes twice a day. On my "month off," I inhale a different antibiotic through a podhaler. This is a simple cylindrical device that I insert a capsule tablet into, press a button to puncture it, and then inhale the tablet's powder contents. I repeat this three times, and in total using a podhaler takes about two minutes twice a day. It also requires no washing up, making it ideal for my busy schedule and poor domestic skills. Even on my month off, however, I still nebulise two lots of mucus clearing aids (mucolytics). The first, hypertonic saline, is a salty solution that helps loosen secretions, therefore helping the mucus to be coughed out. This takes 15 minutes every day. The other, dornase alfa, cuts through the debris left behind after lung bug battles and takes only 3 minutes to inhale. Despite it's speedy inhalation time, it needs to be done an hour before physio, making it more of a logistical challenge to fit in than it initially appears.

I kept saying I would take time off to rest from the madness of commuting, but the constant worry that work would dry up meant I answered every availability email with a resounding YES! The constant exposure to new bugs was also taxing, indeed I don't think I was cold free once in the 5 years I commuted. As a result, my lung function began to dip a little, and after a few different emergency oral antibiotic courses, my doctors decided I need to take the plunge and have my first lot of IVs.

My first experience as an inpatient needing IVs was 2013. By that point I was 22 years old, and avoiding hospitalisation for an exacerbation (flare up of lung infection) up to that point had been quite a feat. By the time most CF patients have reached adulthood they will usually have had a lot of IV experience, with many on regular two-week courses every 2-4 months. Although I wasn't really unwell, my lung function had dropped, suggesting that I wasn't fighting my lung bugs quite as well as I needed to. CF patients usually need IVs very regularly, either to try and kill new bugs before they take hold, or to stop long term bugs from getting too powerful. It's good to think of IVs as being like the heavy artillery in the ongoing battle of the lungs. The very first line of defence is physiotherapy. By using different breathing techniques, mucus can be dislodged from the tubes in the lungs and moved up and out. In most people, the mucus is the body's natural defence – trapping bugs and stopping them from becoming infections. However, cystic fibrosis mucus is so sticky that even with physiotherapy it can't always be shifted, and so the bugs get settled in and start to party. At this point, oral antibiotics are introduced to try and stop the bugs getting too cosy. If this doesn't work then the big guns are brought in, and IVs are used. Now unfortunately CF bugs are tough cookies, and not easy to get rid of. If the bugs cannot be killed then the patient becomes "colonised" and a combination of nebulised and oral antibiotics are taken daily to try and reduce the symptoms and stop the nasty things becoming too much. Eventually lung infections will become too overwhelmming, but this can take quite a long time.

I went into the hospital to have a two-week course of IVs in the March. I took the time off work, and braced myself ready. Going into hospital for IVs when you are not desperately ill is a strange concept. Firstly, although the IVs are very important, the hospital staff must prioritise those patients who are seriously unwell first for beds. This makes complete sense, but as CF units are generally small and patients can become desperately unwell at very short notice, there is no way to get an exact date until the day itself. This is fine for a person with no dependents, but now I have three children to organise last minute childcare for it is quite frustrating. That being said I try to remind myself whenever I do need to come in that I should be grateful for this uncertainty and waiting– after all, at least I'm not needing to come in immediately because my health has suddenly deteriorated dangerously. For this reason, home IVs are a good compromise. They allow patients to continue to live normal lives whilst doing their treatments, and stops the risk of additional infections whilst in hospital. Or at least, live as normally as possible allowing for at least three half hour breaks in the day to mix up and then self-inject a number of high strength antibiotics and anti-sickness drugsx. I have done quite a few courses of home IVs, but as an adult with no one relying on me they are hard work, and with three tiny children they are nigh on impossible, and so my team would therefore rather I come in and have my IVs so that I can have some rest and extra physiotherapy at the same time. I also have a continuous IV drug called aminophylline nowadays, but that's another story. Home IVs require the patient to mix up their own medications and then administer them through either a line or a port into their own bloodstream. I have long lines, which look like the little cannulas you might see in the back of a person's hand in a hospital, but they extend from 8 to 22cm under the skin and usually sit somewhere between the wrist and the shoulder. This sounds horrendous, and the very first time I administered IVs to myself through my line I did have to have a little lie down afterwards, but actually like most things they become normal remarkably quickly. Obviously, there is an infection risk with having a line that leads straight into a vein, and care needs to be taken not to knock or dirty the site. It's also important that the line doesn't become blocked as it will need to be replaced which is a pain. I've only once had a line last the full two weeks of IVs as my veins collapse (or "blow") with the strain, and therefore I need to come into the hospital during the IV period to have a new line. I also need to come in to have bloods to check the doses of antibiotics aren't too high as some antibiotics can have nasty long-term side effects if they are too high. Tobramycin, for example, can lead to ringing in the ears and eventually deafness. My liver levels tend to go up during a course of IVs, and this is monitored as well. On a less serious but rather horrible note, IVs also make me tired, nauseous and upset my stomach to an almost apocalyptic level. This isn't really a surprise though. After all, IV antibiotics are the drug equivalent of nuclear war heads for the insides, and so side effects are inevitable.

My first hospital stay was a peculiar experience. I went in for two weeks, but actually left on day ten, completing the final four days of the intravenous antibiotic course by administering them to myself at home. Until this point I had always assumed that hospital admissions would be as the result of severe illness, and therefore I would spend the time lying in bed, too poorly to do anything. In reality, this is not the case at all. My hospital stays have, so far, always been pre-emptive treatments, aiming to boost back up slipping lung function, helping me gain that ever-elusive weight and generally giving me a chance to rest and re-cooperate when the pressures of normal life have caused me to lose focus on my health. Twice they have also been to help boost me ready for minor operations. This is all "normal", and therefore the biggest difficulty of a hospital stay is actually ordeal by boredom. Cross-infection risks (combined with practicality) means I end up just sitting in a room for two weeks. Nurses and housekeepers ply me with food, and every few hours someone pops in to take my observations (OBs – blood pressure, temperature, pulse and oxygen saturation levels). A TV is supplied, but I mostly just read. When I go to hospital nowadays I pack a large bag with a few changes of clothes, then cram half a library into the remaining space. I once tried adult colouring, but that was an error. Dullness on top of dullness. The staff tell me about their CF patients who are in for months at a time, which makes me feel horrible for them, and guiltily grateful that I'm only doing two weeks. It's not that long in the grand scheme of things really. But it's not all bad. The staff are all friendly, and the more I go in the more faces become familiar. I see the same nurses again and again, learning about their families, their housing issues and their feelings on Brexit. The boredom is punctuated with different staff popping in every few hours to ask questions, bring cups of tea (and Calshakes), perform physiotherapy and watch me ride an exercise bike, and I chat to all of them. The cleaners moan about the nurses, the nurses gripe about the doctors and the housekeepers roll their eyes at the health care assistants.

Over time I have gotten used to the boredom and just try to enjoy the little quirks of the hospital and its staff. During one stay a HCA, brand new to the job, employed an inventive new take on cross infection policy. He pulled his tea trolley up outside my room, banged on the door and hollered, "TEA, COFFEE OR HOT CHOCOLATE, DARLING?" without opening the door. I'd never been offered hot chocolate before, so I plumped for that option. There was a pause, and a slight jangling of cups. Clearly, he didn't have the means for making hot chocolate. Unperturbed he called back through the door: "NO PROBLEM! I'LL JUST BE A MINUTE!" I was impressed by his dedication to his new job as I heard him leave the trolley and head off to scour the hospital for hot chocolate at 9pm on a Saturday night. He returned a whole 20 minutes later and shoved a steaming mug through the tiniest of cracks in the door, leaving it on the floor for me to collect. I shouted "THANKYOU!!" back, even though the door was neither thick nor soundproof, and heard him rattling off down the corridor, stopping to shout through other doors, the choice of hot chocolate no longer being proffered. He was so eager he did his round again at 5am, but unsurprisingly there were no takers.

Cleaners and housekeepers are deeply important staff members for a long-term patient. They hold the key to everything, know what's going on with everyone and love to chat, which when you've been incarcerated for even just a few days is a breath of fresh air. Housekeepers are also able to supply additional juice and occasionally whole fresh fruit, which when everyone else is ramming high fat food and drinks at you is a much-needed relief.

It's hard to keep up with the vast amount of eating required during a stay. At home, I can force a lot of food in. I'm always spinning so many plates, even the postman commenting that my hands are "a bit full" one day whilst helping me chase the errant dog down the road AGAIN, that I burn the calories I'm eating. During a hospital stay, however, I just sit around feeling horribly full for most of the two weeks.

The doctors are split into two categories – the juniors run around like headless chickens, clutching their ward papers and making endless notes and to-do lists. I recognise the exhausted expressions of my own doctor friends and always want to tell them to come in and have a sneaky sit down, but that's probably inappropriate. I imagine they'd be too busy anyway. The consultants, on the other hand, generally look relaxed and on top of life. I'm sure they are just as busy and stressed as everyone else, the NHS being overstretched in every direction, but they give the appearance of complete calm. The only clue to the hectic nature of their work schedules is that they never actually appear to leave the hospital.

The psychological toll of inpatient stays on a patient as healthy as I am is hard to explain. On the one hand, I get irritated about having to come in, grumpily plotting escape before my red allergy wristband has even been fastened, I'm so desperate to just be left to live a normal life. I have to temper this by reminding myself that if I don't go in and have my IVs I will be kissing my normal life goodbye a lot sooner than I should. But on the other hand, when I am in and sat feeling frustrated and bored, usually texting my husband and best friend so they know just how bored I am, I feel guilty because I know that just down the corridor there will most likely be someone with CF my age or even younger desperately trying to breathe, fighting for life, who would probably give their right arm for "boredom" to be their biggest problem right now. Although I don't enjoy being in the hospital, it is important to remember that, comparatively speaking, I am having an easy time of being there. I am acutely conscious of the fact that one day I will need to go to hospital because I am seriously unwell, and then I will look back on the weeks when I used to go in for pre-emptive treatments and roll my eyes at how grudging I was.

The only time I have been too unwell to be bored was during a stay where I reacted badly to the drugs I was being given. I was incredibly sick and constantly nauseous, unable to eat and losing weight hand over fist as a result; a situation not helped by the earnest and kind-hearted housekeeper leaving a full English breakfast at my bedside at 8am every morning – removing it at 11 with a disappointed sigh, well after the smell of egg had permeated the room entirely. Over the eight days I was given the medications the nurses became increasingly militant, angrily asking me to confirm my allergies before each dose, at first muttering under their breaths, but eventually openly and aggressively commenting how ridiculous they felt the treatment was. The treatment was a combination of intravenous drugs – three antibiotics, Septrin, Tazocin and meropenem, with a continuous drip of aminophylline for good measure.

Aminophylline is a type of bronchodilator, which means it that it opens the airways up by relaxing the chest muscles and increasing the contractions of the diaphragm. When combined with physiotherapy this makes it easier to cough out the plugs of mucus that are blocking the tubes in the lungs (bronchioles). It's very clever, and combined with the other heavy antibiotics the hope is to beat my lung bugs into submission. The combination proved effective – my lung function jumped up to 85% - but, unfortunately, I was allergic to at least three of the medications and reacted by being horribly sick. The doctor prescribed three different types of anti-sickness to try and ease the symptoms, but although they took the edge off I was still too nauseous to eat or even read. My bag of books remained untouched, the pages of the one I tried to read swimming in front of my eyes. My best friend, a doctor at another hospital, whistled slightly when I recounted my experience to her, commenting that my doctors had given me "the full domestos treatment". The consultant looked ever so slightly more confused every time she came in as the dose was actually too low to be clinically effective, and therefore my reaction seemed disproportionate. I did feel slightly sorry for her, hoping the nurses weren't being as hostile to her as they were claiming to be. What medicines should be given and at what dose isn't clear cut for any illness, especially one as complex as CF. I always think fighting cystic fibrosis is an attitude of mind. It's trench warfare from the very beginning, with most treatments offering only small victories, most of which are difficult to measure, against a relentless, unbeatable enemy.

My first time as an inpatient showed me a different side of CF. My nurses were all lovely, and commented every time they saw me how wonderful it was to have a cystic fibrosis patient in their early 20s who had no prior inpatient or even IV experience. They were pleased to have someone "so well" and made a huge fuss over me. This was very kind of them, but left me feeling a little cold inside. It's hard to explain to people who don't have a chronic condition what it's like to have something but not really be too affected by it. I felt a strange sense of both sadness and worry, which was twinged with a low level of guilt. Sadness at the knowledge that the other patients were so ill, and the worry that this will eventually happen to me. It's easy for me to close my mind to the suffering that other CF patients go through. We aren't allowed to meet, and so I don't actually know first-hand how the condition is taking its toll on others. My only real insight into how other patients are doing comes from brief sightings in the distance – sometimes in the car park, occasionally passing at pharmacy- half smiling, half trying to move away as quickly as possible.

As the bug specific clinics are always on the same days I see the same people from time to time, and can see that the other patients are looking more tired, thinner and occasionally one has added oxygen to their needs. My first experience as an inpatient, however, opened my eyes to how lonely a condition it is. The nurses commented how wonderful it was that I had a visitor come every day, and my husband came every evening. Most CF patients don't get that, they said. It's so normal to be in hospital so far from home for so long that families can't manage to visit every day, and friends start to dwindle. I was horrified by one nurse telling me the girl in the room down the corridor had been in 6 weeks, and not one person had visited her the entire time. She was a good 18 months younger than me, making her only 20.

After nearly two weeks, the nurses had trained me up enough that I was released into the world to finish the course at home. This brief experience of hospital got rid of my pent-up anger towards the design industry for refusing to give me a full-time job. I went to hospital with the crazy idea that I could just continue working remotely whilst having my IVs. This proved impossible – IVs make me very tired and quite nauseous, and inpatient life is so out of sync with real life that running my time to business hours was just not possible. Although I was not (and am still not) a regular inpatient, the knowledge that this could become a regular thing would be an understandably off-putting point for a small studio when they are looking at a large number of candidates.

Although inpatient stays have never been too regular for me, visits for shorter periods of time are so normal to me that I had never really thought about their frequency until I started work. It was only then that I realised that asking to have an afternoon off every month or so for a jolly to the hospital was actually quite an unusual thing to do.

Hospitals, to most people, are frightening places with strange beeps and scary machines. I find them to be strangely restful. They're quiet, everyone is nice and there's something fascinating about watching a whole world of staff and patients go about their busy days from the quiet vantage of the waiting room. Not, to be fair, that I see many waiting rooms nowadays. Cross infection rules are so strict that most appointments are spent sat in a side room with staff coming to see me. For most patients, hospitals are a world where time is suspended, normal everyday worries are left outside and they are just left with the thought of the next test; fearing diagnosis and the anxiety of a prognosis. For me, a long-term patient who grew up around hospitals, but has never yet been seriously unwell, I don't have these worries. I'm not waiting on a diagnosis, prognosis has been long established and every test is just check up to see how good or bad things are looking. Obviously, there are a multitude of places I'd rather be, but as long as it's just a short day trip, I don't really mind being in one.

Annual review days, or MOTs, in particular are just a chance to sit quietly by myself in a warm room with a book, thinking my own thoughts. Admittedly someone arrives to stab me every now and again, and I do have to fill in a few slightly baffling questionnaires, but it's not the worst way to spend a morning and early afternoon. Despite only lasting about 5 hours there is always both a scheduled snack and lunch break, just to make sure all calorific opportunities have been suitably seized. The term "snack break" is something of a misnomer for a non-CF patient though; last time the nurse supplied me with two bags of crisps and three chocolate bars. This was lovely, but I imagine a uniquely CF situation. On these days, I see a member of every part of the CF team and chat about how the last twelve months have been. This allows the whole team to get together and make any plans for the next 12 months, and the results and any follow up are then relayed to me at my next clinic appointment. But other than these small chats and a scan or two to make sure none of my organs are sneakily breaking faster than they should be, they are (especially since the children came along) calm affairs, and given the choice between an annual review on my own and a morning at a loud, sticky soft play, I know which I'd opt for. Of course, there are always exceptions to every rule. During an MOT day whilst pregnant with my twins a miscommunication amongst the nursing staff meant my GTT was delayed, and ended up being done late on in the morning.

Glucose Tolerance Tests (GTTs) are the best way to tell if a patient has developed diabetes or not. Diabetes goes hand in hand with cystic fibrosis as the production of mucus, combined with inflammation, in the pancreas often causes the insulin ducts to block. This stops insulin being correctly supplied into the small intestine, resulting in CFRD, or cystic fibrosis related diabetes. This doesn't happen to every patient, but as better treatment is leading to patients living longer despite their lung disease, CFRD is on the increase. For a GTT, a patient fasts for between eight and twelve hours, then has a blood test done whilst fasting. They then drink an extremely glucose rich drink, called Polycal, and have another blood test two hours later, at which point they are able to break their fast. The blood tests allow doctors to see if the body metabolises glucose correctly, as the presence of diabetes would stop this from happening.

Normally I am asked to fast from midnight, and the annual review appointment begins at 8am with the first bloods. This time exhaustion from pregnancy had caused me to go to bed at 8pm the night before, and nurses didn't start taking the first bloods until 10 the next morning. This was fine, but did mean that at 6 months pregnant with twins I went without food and drink for 16 hours. Hospital staff who specialise in CF are always extremely generous with food, eager to ram in any extra calories wherever they can. The CF nurse who came to check in on me was no exception to this rule, and was horrified to discover I hadn't eaten for so long. He raced off to the hospital restaurant, declaring that the usual post GTT sandwich and cup of tea simply would not do. On his return, he brought with him an impressively over stacked plate, piled high with a somewhat bizarre combination of foods. Chuffed with himself, he informed me that he had pleaded with the restaurant staff to give his pregnant, wasting away patient both the leftovers from the full English they'd served for breakfast plus a hearty portion of chips and a decent sized gravy oozing pie for good measure. He declared it was "Blunch", as it was far too big for an ordinary brunch. I was impressed by both his ability to convince the restaurant staff to part with so much food, and his economical attitude towards washing up, having chosen to combine both meals on one plate. I thanked him, and he raced off, presumably to shove food into other unsuspecting patients. As hungry as I was, and as kind as it was for him to supply me with so much, I will confess I was overwhelmed at the sight of 4 sausages, 3 bacon rashers, scrambled eggs, four halved tomatoes, a copious amount of beans, a big pie and a glut of chips all vying for centre stage on the plate. I dug in, but quickly began to flag, the presence of two stomach-squashing babies not helping the situation. The nurse popped back to check I was ok, looking ever so slightly crestfallen at my slow progress. I smiled another thank-you and he left again, promising to return in a bit for my plate. I did my best, but barely made a dent in the mound. He seemed so eager to please, and, determined not to hurt his feelings, I momentarily suffered from a misplaced sense of maternal instinct, doubtlessly brought on by raging hormones. Instead of admitting my defeat, I sneakily made a nest of Clinell wipes from the handy box next to my head in the bottom of my handbag, and tipped most of the meat pie, two sausages, the bacon and a good quantity of beans and egg in on top. Obviously, this was a gross misuse of NHS supplies, but I was desperate not to upset the bloke. I'd just clipped my bag shut, silently cursing it's lack of zip, when he reappeared, expressing his delight that I'd put so much away, the plate being clear bar a number of chips. "Wow! Abi! I really didn't think you'd manage even half of that, it was MASSIVE!" I'd already realised I'd made a grave error of judgement, and this just compounded that feeling. He left, jokily promising to put in a good word with the dietitian for me, leaving me sat next to a working radiator on a hot July day, with an already smelly pile of food hidden in a bag below my chair.

The appointment continued. The dietitian had indeed been informed of my mammoth efforts and incredible appetite, and she spent an awkward few moments praising me for all the hard work I was putting in, despite the obvious hindrance of foetal twins. I surreptitiously spread my skirt wide to try and hide the offending bag, guiltily accepting her praise. Fortunately, my pregnancy meant that I did not have to hang around for a CT Scan or Ultrasound, which was a huge relief, as the smell of egg was already pervading the bag. It was probably my imagination, but I'm sure the pharmacist had been slightly holding her breath as she went through my medications.

The day ward nurse came over to tell me I could go, and I jumped up delightedly. The nurse saw my bag and bent down. "Here you are sweetheart, let me reach that for you," she said. "Nope!" I all but shouted, almost knocking her flying in my rush to grab my bag and hold it shut so she couldn't see the grotesque pile of food sat in it. She looked at me with a rather less friendly expression and I left as quickly as possible, clutching the bag tightly to me.

When I got home the combination of collecting Ben from nursery, signing for a neighbour's parcel and letting the dog out caused me to forget that my bag was sat in the porch, unemptied. When John arrived home from work that night he demanded to know what the horrendous stench was as he opened the door. I tried to explain why I'd felt the need to smuggle a large quantity of food out of a hospital in a particularly nice handbag, but however much I elucidated to him that I would hate to upset an extremely nice nurse, he rolled his eyes at my madness and, oblivious to my hormonally unbalanced condition, even went so far as to suggest that the man would "probably have survived". I ended up having to throw the bag away as, despite several washes, it's inside never quite recovered from the onslaught of food juices and antiseptic chemicals it had been subjected to.

-5-

THE MARATHON

Before my first hospital stay and IVs, I had feared them coming for a long time. I was sure that it would be a horrendous experience, a sign that the wind had changed, leaving me at lower lung function, changing how my life would be lead from then on. This was not realised and I therefore left feeling high on life, no longer worn down with the exhaustion that comes of commuting and happy with my newly regained higher lung function. I had gone into hospital at the end of a dull, gloomy March, and came out into a warm April. It felt as though spring had sprung overnight, and I was optimistic for the future.

The first weekend I was out I watched the coverage of the London Marathon and, like any good armchair athlete, proclaimed that I could easily do that. Now I am not a natural runner, but I was feeling invincible and, inspired by the race, I nipped out for a run of my own that afternoon.

Exercise is a hugely important part of CF. First and foremost, it's a form of physiotherapy as it makes the lungs work harder, encouraging deep breaths which helps loosen mucus, therefore keeping lungs healthy. Muscle tone is also important as over time malabsorption can cause malnutrition, including a lack of calcium, resulting in weakened bones. Eventually CF patients can develop osteoporosis, and muscle tone helps keep weak bones protected. On top of this arthritis due to the inflammation caused by the body's immune system responding to infections a bit too heavily is also common, and exercise can help to ease these symptoms. Finally, a healthy heart is always important in a condition where oxygen supply will become scarce, and the heart will need to work harder to make up for it.

I was pleased to find that my life long obsession with exercise rendered a 5k relatively easy for me and, blinded with an almost manic level of self-belief, wrote an impassioned letter to the Cystic Fibrosis Trust explaining why I would be a perfect fit for their running team and worthy of a place in the following year's marathon. A wiser person than myself would probably have balked at the thought of running a marathon with such little experience, after all there's quite a difference between a casual 5km jog and a 44km run, but I'm rashly optimistic about life generally and didn't really see it being a problem. I spent the next week or so running, then life, and work, got back into full swing. John and I began to pass like ships in the night again, and I promptly forgot all about my foolhardy proclamation.

Seven months later, at the beginning of November, on a cold Saturday morning, I received a letter through the door, congratulating me on securing my place in the London Marathon and explaining that my gold bond slot required a minimum of £2,000 sponsorship money. My initial reaction at reading this was just to laugh and I ran to the garage to compliment John on his excellent practical joke. He quickly put me to right, and I'm afraid my response to learning that I had in fact committed to running 26.2 miles with minimal time to train whilst also raising a large sum of cash, is, unfortunately, unprintable. My parents, barely hiding their amusement, bought me some trainers as an early Christmas present, and I set off running as much as possible in training.

The winter of 2013-2014 was long, cold and very, very wet. I spent hours jogging, hating CF, myself for my poorly thought out ambition, mud and any other runner who dared look happy at wading through said mud. I had a brief break in training during the December when a minor reaction to 5 weeks of ciprofloxacin gave me tendonitis, but after two weeks off the pain in my shins righted itself, and I got back to it.

Fortunately, being a freelancer meant I was able to work flexible hours and as the marathon date drew nearer I was able to take time off to complete the long runs. By March the weather had broken, I'd discovered my stride and, unbelievably, found myself becoming one of those hateful people who actually enjoys running. I was covering the long runs easily and even silently dared to dream of a reasonable time of approximately four and a half hours. Fundraising was also going fantastically well. My friends, family and co-workers all dug deep and sponsored me very generously. Mostly, it must be said, out of sheer disbelief that a person would not only enter a marathon with both a serious medical condition and no prior running experience, but could also then forget about said undertaking. A few people vaguely suggested a smaller race would probably have been a better starting point, which is completely true, but I'm an impulsive person who can't ever do things by half.

All too soon the weekend of the marathon arrived and John and I packed ourselves off to London, staying overnight on the Saturday in preparation. We went out for a reasonably late dinner so I could carb load ready for the big event. Unfortunately, my nerves got the better of me and I massively underestimated the amount of Creon my high fat and carb meal required.

Sunday 13th April 2014 was a beautiful, sunny day. I put on my running kit, including a Cystic Fibrosis Trust tee shirt emblazoned with my name, stuck my marathon number on and, with some trepidation, walked to the nearest tube stop, experiencing a bizarre new side of London on the way. People smiled and called "good luck!", TFL workers opened gates for me and random strangers offered me their seats on the tube. Although my nerves were high I began to relax into this new, enjoyable underground situation, vaguely wondering whether I could get away with wearing my vest and number for my commute on the Monday morning.

All too soon, however, I joined the crowd at Greenwich Park. This was a surreal experience – a huge mass of lycra clad people stretching their limbs on the grass, interspersed with a surprisingly large number of fancy dress characters and a man with an actual fridge strapped to his back. I went to my starting pen and started to lightly warm up. When a person is unfortunate enough to secure a spot in the London Marathon they are asked to fill in a form estimating their approximate finishing time. As my form arrived at a time when I was not anticipating having to trudge through 26.2 miles, I had no idea of how long it would take me to travel such a distance, or even how long people normally take. I therefore panicked and guessed at 9 hours. Undeniably, this was a ridiculously long time to put – even fridge man did it in 6 hours 11 minutes and 57 seconds – but it meant that the organisers had carefully put me at the very back, amongst all the over achievers in humungously heavy costumes. I actually felt like I'd struck gold – how can a person be nervous about running 26.2 miles when they've got Big Bird, a pantomime horse (both ends!) and a man with a fridge around them? We chatted about our chosen charities for a bit and soon we were off.

By 10:30 am I had crossed the starting line and was gently settling into the swing of it. The sun, which at 9 am was pleasantly warm, had revealed its true colours and the temperature was steadily rising. By 11 the marathon organisers had already turned on showers for people to run through to get relief from the heat. For me all was going smoothly. I'd left behind all of the more outlandish fancy dress wearers and was slowly but steadily moving my way forward through the pack. I passed the Cutty Sark at a good pace, waving at my family as I went. At the Tower of London, the halfway point a mere 13 miles in (ha! 13 miles. Ridiculous!) I was bang on time for my four-and-a-half-hour allowance and feeling good. By mile 14, however, things were very different.

Cystic fibrosis, despite popular opinion, is not, in fact, "just a lung thing." The mucus that builds up in the tubes in the lungs is also building up in the other organs of the body. Particularly the pancreas, small intestine and liver. These are slowly blocking up with the same mucus, although of course this time nothing can be coughed out. Instead the tubes of the body just block up over time. This is particularly true in the pancreas. The pancreas, as organs go, seems to be somewhat overlooked by most. It's the oft forgotten organ that's actually responsible for an awful lot, specifically the supply of enzymes for digestion and hormones for insulin production and management.

When anyone eats any food, they begin to break it down and digest it as soon as it goes into their mouth with their saliva. As the food travels down the oesophagus the saliva stays with it, slowly breaking it down. The food goes into the stomach where it is broken up further by stomach acids, and then passes out into the small intestine. Here the pancreas passes enzymes down tubes called pancreatic ducts into the small intestine, allowing the broken-down food to be split into its basic components and the nutrients absorbed through the intestinal walls. The intestinal tubes are lined with little folds called villi. These are covered with tiny little hairs called microvilli, and the combination of the two hugely increases the surface area of the intestines, allowing nutrients to be absorbed as well as possible. Both the intestines and the pancreatic ducts are tubes, and predictably they are lined with epithelial cells. This means that in a CF patient the water and salt are not able to pass correctly, and so the mucus in both is thicker. In the pancreas, this means that the pancreatic enzymes do not flow correctly. The tubes block up, and so the enzymes are unable to get to the small intestine.

Cystic fibrosis requires a person to eat huge amounts of fat, partially because we are unable to digest fat or absorb the nutrients properly through our intestines, but also because we require so many calories to fight our lung bugs. We are also expected to exercise as much as possible to help with said lung issues, thus we burn through all the calories we do manage to get from our food very quickly. The irony of a condition that necessitates the consumption of so much fat, whilst simultaneously denying the sufferer the ability to actually absorb it, is not lost on me.

Creon is a replacement enzyme, taking the place of the enzymes unable to travel down the pancreatic ducts, and allows us to digest fat. Now Creon is wonderful stuff, taken very gratefully by a lot of CF patients. Even the least compliant of patients won't be caught without a pot of it on their person. It breaks down the fat and nutrients in the food, allowing them to be absorbed through the walls of the small intestine. Although Creon works well, it's not 100% effective and so, over time, the walls of the intestines start to scale up with undigested fat. The combination of mucus secretions and undigested fat in the small intestine means that over time the tubes get thinner and thinner, and the surface area for absorbing nutrients shrinks. The secretions can cause inflammation, which also thins the tubes. If a person doesn't take their Creon correctly, even for just one meal, this results in undigested food needing to make its way through the intestines to where it can *ahem* exit the body. When combined with the other issues of swelling and inflammation, the result is a large mass and a tiny tube. I think we can all tell that this is going to go wrong.

And indeed, it does. Constipation is a regular problem in CF, as the mucus normally used in the intestines as a lubricant to help move poo through the system is stickier. Not to be too graphic, it's like trying to go down a slide with or without washing up liquid. This problem is treated with basic laxatives, and at first doesn't sound too bad. Over time, however, the constant excess fat being left in the digestive system mixes with all the sticky mucus causing blockages to form in the small intestine. This is called Distal Intestinal Obstruction Syndrome (DIOS). Although it has similarities with constipation, it is a very different beast. Normally, constipation happens in the bowel. I'm sure you will know it is painful, as it is most likely you will have experienced it at some point, but it can be dealt with relatively easily. In DIOS, the blockage is not just poo, but sticky mucus and undigested food. It occurs in the small intestine, usually near the end of a section called the ileum, which means the blockage needs to travel all the way through the rest of the large intestine and bowel before relief can be had. And, most importantly, the blockage can often be fused to the wall of the intestine by the horribly sticky mucus. Blockages can happen higher up in the small intestine, but fortunately these are not quite so common.

I have only once had the start of a bowel blockage. I was prescribed a bottle of liquid medicine called Gastrografin. The consultant prescribing it asked if I'd had it before. When I said no, she grimaced slightly and told me to go home, clear my social schedule for the weekend, then hold my nose and drink it. I laughed.

 I wasn't laughing later.

If home treatments are not working, the patient is often forced to go in to the hospital to have their bowel blockage sorted. They are given seriously strong laxatives and pain relief. Frequently the laxatives are poured in through an NG tube (or through a PEG if there is one) and if that's still not working through an enema. Eventually the situation will be sorted, but this can take time. Sometimes days, sometimes longer.

You might think that this agonising situation should be remedied quickly with a small surgical procedure. Unfortunately, this isn't the recommended way. Once DIOS has occurred, it will keep reoccurring. Cutting into a person to remove a blockage once wouldn't be brilliant, especially when you consider just how broken the mucus crusted CF digestive system already is, but to keep cutting into them would be disastrous. Instead patients are given regular laxatives to help the situation before it happens, and need to keep as hydrated as possible at all times to try and keep things moving. There are times when there is no other option but to perform surgery, although fortunately this is not too common.

It is important to note that not all CF patients are pancreas insufficient. For some reason, some people (between 10-15% of CF patients) are able to pass enzymes down their pancreatic ducts and therefore digest fat like anyone else. They still need to eat more than the average person as they are still burning a lot more energy fighting lung bugs and exercising so much, but they don't need to take Creon as well. You could be forgiven for thinking that these patients have got off scot free, but that's not really fair. Although they might not have to bother with Creon, these people still have epithelial cells in their pancreas like everyone else. This means there are still problems that are caused by their cystic fibrosis as the salt and water are still not being passed correctly. These people are prone to pancreatitis (although not everyone who is pancreas sufficient will have this problem), which is a nasty complication whereby the pancreas mismanages the enzymes and actually beings to digest itself. Although this can be treated it is still horribly painful. A small, particularly unlucky, number of pancreas insufficient CF patients have been reported to have had pancreatitis as well, but it is rarer.

As one of the more common pancreas insufficient CF sufferers, I spent quite a lot of time in my school library researching exactly what the pancreas is and how the intestines work, or at least how mine should have worked. Of course, reading is all well and good, but having no one to share my learnings with meant that I accrued a large biological vocabulary that I may have understood, but sadly could not pronounce. I was made painfully aware of this once when dozing off at the back of a biology class. The teacher, spotting my glazed eyes and slack jaw, called my name out, pointing at a handy diagram of the body on the wall next to her. "Abi! Wake up! What's this?" She was pointing at the middle of the small intestine, and in snapping awake I called back "it's the Jelly Juno Mum!" Much merriment ensued, and it took quite a while for my classmates to let me forget my odd answer, certain as they were that I'd made the fatal error of calling a teacher "Mum". I had actually been attempting to say jejunum, which is the bit of the intestine where absorption of nutrients begins.

Mismanaging Creon for just one meal results in a deeply painful cramping sensation, as the intestines grumble at having to force the undigested fat through tiny tubes. I know I've messed up my Creon because I feel a sharp, burning pain in my abdomen and break out in an uncontrollable cold sweat. If I've really gone wrong I usually end up lying in bed in the foetal position, cursing food, life and anyone in the vicinity before eventually needing to race to the toilet. Sadly, when one has both eaten enough for two meals and is 14 miles into a 26.2 mile race that's not really an option, and so I kept on running, even picking my pace up in a crazy attempt to get to the end quick enough to deal with this hellish situation in peace. By 17 miles, however, I could run no further and began walking, then doubled over hobbling, to the finish.

After some time, I had dropped back far enough that the lycra clad runners had become fancy dress wearers, then crazy fancy dress runners, then, finally, at about mile 23, fridge man overtook me. I was now amongst the walking injured, a truly depressing place to be. Marathon stewards began to lean in to me from the side asking me if I was ok. More than one tried to insist that I stopped. I refused, grimacing at them and pushing on towards the finish. To be fair, I was sweaty, shaking, holding my stomach and looking pretty miserable. The combination of heat, pain and exertion had covered me in tiny salt crystals from my evaporated sweat. Even by 20+ mile marathon runner standards, I looked rough. Fortunately, however, it was late enough in the day that the carnival atmosphere of the crowd had well and truly taken over. Strangers shouted "Abi! Abi! Abi!" as I passed and more than one offered me a can of alcohol, declaring it looked more beneficial to me than the more standard jelly baby. Boyed by the ridiculous nature of the crowd, I asked a steward just how far I'd gone. Surprised, he pointed ahead to Big Ben and told me there was only a mile left. The thought of ending this horror (and, I'll admit, finding a toilet) spurred me on and I ran the final mile as fast as I could, dodging round other runners, sprinting down the mall and over the line. It had taken me a whopping 5 hours and 35 minutes, but I was done. I met my family at horse guards parade. They wanted to take photos. I wanted to lie down. Eventually we found a cold patch of empty pavement amongst the crowds and I lay down on my stomach and cried.

All in all, it was not the most successful experience in my life, and definitely one of the more unpleasant. But over £5000 was raised for the CF Trust and I can now forever boast that I once travelled 26.2 miles on foot, which, let's be honest, is why most people run marathons anyway.

-6-

GROWING THE FAMILY

For us, becoming a family of five happened both very slowly and very quickly. We had always talked about wanting children. Indeed, my husband had himself tested for the cystic fibrosis gene a year or so before we were even engaged. We knew we wanted children, but we were not willing to risk giving them CF. Fortunately his test came back negative for the 20 most common genetic mutations, making the chances of having a child with the condition extremely unlikely.

Cystic fibrosis is a genetic condition, which means that it is passed to a child through their parents. Importantly, it is a recessive genetic disease. This means that a person who carries the gene will not have cystic fibrosis. Only a person with two CF genes, one from each parent, will have it. My children all carry a gene, as do my parents and one of my brothers. My other brother carries no gene, having inherited both of my parents non-

CF genes. This makes him the exact opposite of me, who has inherited both of my parent's faulty genes. Now CF, although rare, is actually the most common inherited genetic disorder, and it is estimated that one in twenty-five Caucasians carry the faulty gene.

After we had been married for a few years I began to have a slight dip in my health, and for the first time in my life I had a couple of courses of IV antibiotics and a hospital stay. The side effects of these drugs, and the large amount of additional oral antibiotics I suddenly found myself taking meant that the pill was less effective, and therefore we privately decided to throw caution to the wind and see where life took us. For 2 years nothing happened, but we were neither sad nor happy about this. We were simply at a stage in life where children would be nice, but I was happy to be using my degree and living my commuter life working in London and John was happy enough to do his work. We bought a house, got a dog and generally enjoyed being a young, carefree married couple.

In 2013 we decided that, actually, a baby would be quite nice. We spoke to my CF team and they cautioned us that it would be a risk to my health, particularly after the baby was born, but gave their blessing. The addition of a baby to anyone is a big strain and causes them to readjust their life to fit in their needy, time consuming tiny human. For someone with CF this is an even bigger adjustment as we are already fitting our lives around treatments and hospital time. This doesn't include the sheer exhaustion babies bring with them. For anyone sleep is an important part of life, but for a person constantly waging war on lung bugs, it is vital. Despite this warning, my doctors were happy enough with my condition and were not too worried about us adding a baby in. They commented, however, that my weight was not high enough and I should aim to improve that before we started trying. They also warned us that high mucus levels can cause some women with CF to be infertile, but that we could seek help for that if nothing was happening. The number of women with CF who have children is relatively low, possibly as a result of many being too ill (a lung function below 60% is considered to be too low for safe pregnancy, although there have been some successful pregnancies reported), combined with some who don't want to risk leaving their children without a mother. This leaves little space for research, but I have read that there is estimated to be a 50/50 chance of cervical mucus being thick enough to cause infertility. This left us in a little dilemma. We knew that we had technically been unsuccessful for two years, but we decided to keep this to ourselves and see what happened. We were slightly concerned that two years had passed, but we put that to the back of our minds and carried on with life. The only difference was that suddenly we were "trying". I tried my hardest to put some more weight on and improve my lung function in preparation for a pregnancy.

During this time I was still commuting, and it was beginning to take its toll. I was always exhausted and generally not looking after myself as well as I should have. As a result, my lungs took a dip and I began to grow some funny bugs. In the September of 2014 I began to feel quite unwell, and my doctors began a somewhat unexpected course of home IVs to help me. As they knew I was hoping to fall pregnant they did a pregnancy test before I began the IVs. I had missed my period a couple of weeks before and was really hopeful that I was pregnant. I'd done my own test, but was hopeful it had been a false negative. Unfortunately, the hospital urine test was negative as well and they began the IVs. I was secretly devastated, having thought that 2 years and 8 months in we had finally managed it, and I sat on a bed in the day ward and cried whilst a slightly confused nurse began the first dose.

However, three weeks later the IVs were over and I was still feeling tired and nauseous. My period still hadn't started, and so I repeated the test. It was a positive. We kept the news to ourselves for a day, then I phoned and shared it with my CF nurse. She was very excited for us, but I felt that the bubble had broken slightly. Most couples are able to keep babies secret for a few months, and a lot of my friends have reminisced about how exciting it was having a secret they could smile about to themselves as a couple. We kept it from our families and friends, but let a whole cohort of medical people in on the secret. I was scheduled in for monthly check ups with my CF team and they contacted the obstetrics team at the hospital I was going to go to. This was not my local hospital, but fortunately it was not much further for me to travel. The doctors (and midwives) at this hospital were excellent and were experienced at working with my team to look after CF mothers. Not that there are many of us, it must be said.

I went to my GP to arrange for a midwife appointment and was scheduled for a dating scan. My GP and I were at odds over the dates and so my first scan was actually at 9 weeks, which was an incredible experience. I am no stranger to ultrasounds, but it felt fantastic to be looking at a tiny human, something I was growing inside me, rather than to be checking that my organs weren't sneakily getting too damaged.

My community midwife, whom I met a week or so after the first dating scan was wonderful, although quickly bowed out of my care. As she made more and more notes in the "Additional Health Problems" section of my maternity notes, she began to look a bit unsure, and when she realised I was going to be seeing an obstetrician and having a scan every month she smiled broadly with relief, stated that she could add nothing and wished me all the best. How wrong she was! I was very grateful to her for being so honest. As I was still working and the number of appointments I was having was growing fast, adding in another appointment seemed somewhat unnecessary.

I went through my pregnancy with very little to write home about. I had been told it would be very hard, and I would at some point get gestational diabetes. Actually, I was an irritatingly happy pregnant woman. I glowed, my hair shone and I even slept well. I only grew a small, neat, stretch mark free bump so maternity clothes looked perfect and no one could even see I was pregnant from behind. (If you're currently pregnant and reading this, fear not. Karma bit me in a big way nine months later, trust me.) I didn't get diabetes, although I did have to do the pin prick tests several times a day to check my blood sugars, and I also had to wait around for quite some time after obstetrician appointments to see the diabetes nurse. These were short, sweet check-ups, mostly spent listening to a very surprised nurse saying "Oh! You don't have diabetes!" My lung function actually improved by a few percent and, although my weight gain wasn't brilliant, by the end I had gained about 9 kg.

The ultrasounds were all going well and my obstetrician decided, at about 34 weeks, that things were going so well we should quit whilst we were ahead and scheduled me for an induction at 37 weeks exactly. 37 weeks can technically be referred to as full term, because every woman's natural gestational period is slightly different. By 37 weeks the foetus is fully formed and spends the remaining few weeks simply gaining weight to help it when it finally enters the world. My obstetrician asked me to schedule a sweep with my community midwife 2 days before I was due to come in for induction, in order to help the process. Sweeps are very simple procedures, where the midwife runs (or sweeps) his or her finger around the cervix. This will hopefully separate the amniotic sac from the cervix, causing the body to release hormones which help bring on labour. Appointment booked, I sat back at home, looking forward to meeting our baby.

About a week and a half before I was due to have my induction I began to suffer the most terrible itching all over my skin. It started off relatively mild, but grew worse and worse every day. Unsure what this was, I attempted to continue as normal. The itching became so severe that I started taking cold showers in the middle of the night to try and ease it. In hindsight, I should have phoned someone sooner, but I was focused on counting down days to my induction and didn't really think a bit of an itch was a problem.

On the Monday morning, I went to see my community midwife for my sweep. She was somewhat perturbed to see me scratching frantically at my reddened, slightly broken skin as I came in and almost instantly diagnosed me as having a severe case of obstetric cholestasis. She phoned through to the hospital and told them to expect me. She did do a quick sweep, explaining what cholestasis was and the associated risks (most importantly still birth) at the same time. Then, almost as an afterthought, she drew some blood. "You won't need this," she said, "its textbook cholestasis, they'll just induce you a little earlier. But if they do want to take blood this will save them a bit of time." I phoned John, slightly panicked, sitting in the car outside the GPs. He left work and we went to the hospital, bag in the boot and blood and notes in my hands.

When we arrived at the hospital we were taken to a room where baby could be monitored. The student midwife was not terribly interested in us, and actually began the CTG (baby heart rate tracer) saying, "this will be nice for you to take home with you in an hour." I tried to emphasise what the community midwife had said, and the risks she had told me about, but the student wasn't really interested. She disappeared for a bit and then, because baby's heart rate was fine, she told us we could go. I objected and insisted on seeing someone more experienced. As much as I hate to kick up a fuss, I was concerned that I was being ignored. An older midwife came and sat down kindly with me, wanting to know what was upsetting me. When I explained about the cholestasis and fear of still birth, she told me not to worry. "Cholestasis is rare. You're unlikely to have it, and especially unlikely to have a still birth." Frustrated I agreed to leave, but I handed my already labelled blood in at the maternity reception desk down the corridor to another midwife, telling a white lie that I'd just been told to ask her to send it to be tested for OC. The midwife barely looked up as she took it and put it in with all the other samples. And so we went home, deflated and very, very itchy.

At 9pm that night, however, I received a phone call from the hospital. My bloodwork was back and I not only had cholestasis, but my liver levels were very high. Measuring liver levels is the best way to diagnose cholestasis, and the higher the liver level the worse the cholestasis is. They told me to get a good night's sleep and come in at 8am the next morning for induction.

That night we lay in bed. But neither of us slept.

We arrived bright and early the next morning all raring to go. It turns out that being induced is a slow process. They booked me in, did a trace and then we waited. I had lunch. We waited. Then finally in the middle of the afternoon a lovely midwife came over to pop in the pessary to begin the induction. She carefully explained I wouldn't feel anything at first, and that it was important not to be disheartened if they had to keep replacing the pessary over the next 24 hours. She was very smiley and keen to assure me that although early induction was a very long-winded process every minute was bringing us closer to holding baby.

Pessary in, we wandered off through the hospital, John giddy at the thought of baby coming soon, me anxious, horribly itchy and slightly uncomfortable.

By the time we'd reached the food court downstairs the slight discomfort had become a horrible cramping sensation. We walked round the shops for about quarter of an hour, then decided to move closer to the induction unit. We stopped in a quiet corridor and I jogged up and down trying to get rid of the tight feeling. At last I decided I needed to go and ask the midwives what was happening – I'd been repeatedly told to expect nothing for hours at least, but only 90 minutes in I couldn't stand still for pain.

When we got to the induction unit the midwives were lovely, but told me not to worry, nothing could possibly be happening yet. Mentally I disagreed strongly, but sat on the oversized beach ball as directed anyway. The other women in the bay had all begun induction at some point during the previous evening and all looked bored. Their husbands were all either catching last minute shut eye or staring blankly into space as the women alternated between pacing and ball bouncing. One said she was "slightly achy" but that was it. I, on the other hand, was panting, sweaty and gripped with pain so bad I actually told John I thought I was allergic to the pessary and probably dying as a result. John didn't really know what to do and kept saying unhelpful things like "don't forget to breathe!" whilst looking round anxiously for a passing midwife. Fortunately, a nice student midwife came over and asked if I minded answering her questions about my CF. She was fascinated by my additional health problems, and keen to learn more for her studies. I agreed and answered her questions as well as I could, but it was getting harder and harder to concentrate on what she was actually saying. After about 10 minutes she stopped to look at me properly, and commented that I looked like I might possibly already be having contractions, despite the induction having only just been started. Bent over the bed and trying not to scream, I was less than impressed about this being only a possibility, and she brought over a CTG to check. I was indeed having intense, continuous contractions. The tracer was moving up to the top and then only getting half way down before spiking back up again. The student expressed her surprise and nipped off to find someone to help. Another midwife appeared with a midwife assistant. They looked at me, glanced at the reading and suggested perhaps a move over to the delivery unit to get some pain relief might be a good idea. By this point all self-control had gone and I was lying on the bed screaming, John standing awkwardly next to me trying to remember what the ante natal class had told him to do. The other women were all staring at me, looking half jealous and half terrified at what was coming for them. This was made comically worse as I was wheeled from induction to delivery, through a waiting area full of pregnant women, who watched me screaming with wide, slightly terrified eyes.

The induction ladies handed me to the delivery midwives who took one quick look and pronounced me to already have reached 10 cm. They were about to change shift, so gave me some gas and air and told me to sit tight. After 5 minutes a midwife came back in to sit with me in case anything changed, but actually she spent most of the time trying to wrestle the gas and air off me whenever she thought I might be about to loosen my grip (she didn't manage it; I was high but not mad) and instead had to resort to merely telling me to slow down on it a bit.

Not long later another midwife and a paramedic doing a refresher course on labour came in, they dimmed the lights and the pushing stage began. Within a surprisingly short amount of time Ben was born, coming out screaming in a gush of blood and waters. My midwife was delighted at how easy it had all been, congratulating us and telling me I was born to give birth. I was still high as a kite, but was pleased all had gone well. Ben was bundled up and handed to John to be cuddled whilst she dealt with the placenta and repaired the damage his fast exit had done. After a few minutes she left and returned with a doctor who put in some stitches for her as they were needed unusually high up inside me. They were friendly and patient, despite me being far too high to lie still properly, and soon all was taken care of. At this point the midwife took Ben from John, told him to go and make his good news phone calls and laid Ben on my chest to feed.

We sat in almost complete darkness, the room feeling peaceful after the noisy violence that is natural childbirth, the midwife gently telling me how to best latch Ben on. He didn't seem at all interested, and after only a few minutes the room began to feel too quiet. The midwife turned the light on to see what was happening and inhaled sharply on seeing that Ben was both blue and silently gulping for air. She sprinted from the room and returned seconds later with a paediatrician. The paediatrician put a SATs monitor on Ben's wrist and foot and directed the midwife to bring the cot over. I didn't see what the SATs were reading, but Ben was pulled unceremoniously out of my hands and run out of the door by midwife and paediatrician, so I can only assume they were not good. They passed John at high speed as he came back in from sharing the good news of Ben's safe delivery with our families, and we spent a terrifying 10 minutes waiting for someone to tell us what had happened.

When the midwife returned she explained that Ben had been rushed to the Neonatal Intensive Care Unit (NICU), and the doctors were working to help him breathe properly. She was calm, reassuring and careful to tell us she'd seen a lot worse, and he was in safe hands.

With the baby gone, we didn't really know what to do with ourselves. We were completely shell shocked by the sudden turn of events. Against all odds my pregnancy and labour had been textbook perfect, yet there we were, sat on a delivery unit without a baby. I had a shower and was asked for a urine sample so they could rule out infection in the womb. And with that we were left alone, the midwife checking in periodically to make sure we were ok. Exhausted by the sheer effort and shock of my under 3 hour labour and subsequent lack of baby I went into a deep sleep, but John paced the room unable to settle. At last, 4 hours later, the midwife woke me up to say we were being sent to the postpartum ward, and were able to visit Ben on the way. Instantly I got out of bed to walk there, asking for directions, but she laughed and gently pushed me into a wheel chair. When we got there, he was in an incubator. He had a tube in his nose, was bathed in blue light and was wearing what looked like gigantic foam skiing goggles to protect his eyes from the light. Most frighteningly he had a huge breathing mask on and there was a bubbling machine next to him moving up and down at the same speed as his chest. The doctor came to meet us, and began to explain that Ben seemed to have damaged his lungs on exit, and they were needing to support him with his breathing. He was also very jaundiced, but as he was technically a little premature that was to be expected. I panicked and asked if this was because he had CF. The doctor was confused, but after I'd explained I had CF, she made a note on her papers and told me not to worry, he'd probably just inhaled fluid in his keenness to join the world.

After saying hello to our little baby, we were taken downstairs to the post-natal ward. The midwife told John to go home and sleep (he got none that night, he was far too wound up) then gave me a hug and put me to bed in a bay in one of the corners, telling me not to worry too much. I woke at 5am the next morning to the sound of crying. A lot of crying. In fact an entire ward of crying babies. Everywhere I looked there were women cuddling tiny noise machines, cooing over them and feeding them. Bereft, I went to the midwife station to ask what was going on with my own baby. The midwife shrugged and told me to go up to NICU and find out for myself. Taken aback, I put on my dressing gown and headed out into the hospital. I had come to the ward in semi darkness at just gone midnight the night before, and therefore had no idea where NICU actually was. I limped off (why does no one warn expecting mothers that immediately postpartum it's almost impossible to walk thanks to the extreme bruising caused by the trauma of childbirth?) eventually spotting a sign for the NICU. Unfortunately, it was pointing up some stairs, but I followed it anyway, desperate to find out what was going on with Ben. After I'd climbed two flights, however, I sat down in the stair well, unable to go any further. I'd given birth less than 10 hours previously and even opening the heavy stair well fire door was now too much effort. Fortunately, a porter came into the stairwell. He was startled to find me sitting there in my pyjamas and asked why I hadn't used the lift right next to the stairwell door. At this I burst into tears and told him in one gabbling sentence that I was looking for NICU to find my poorly baby and I didn't even know where he was, let alone the lifts. He pulled a hanky from his pocket and shushed me gently. He then let me lean on him as we walked up the rest of the stairs and over to the NICU. He then showed me the lifts directly in front of the NICU and told me which floor to get off at to go to the postpartum ward. I saw him again in the lift the next day, and he told me I looked a million times better and hoped baby was doing as well.

When I got to Ben in the NICU he was doing well. Although not much had changed nothing had gotten worse, and his nurse was pleased with him. She asked why I'd walked there as the midwives are supposed to bring recently postpartum women up in wheel chairs if there are no available family members to do so. Since attending toddler groups with Ben I have met a lot of the other mothers who had NICU babies, and learned that my unpleasant experience was far from unique. The NICU staff, understandably, believe their duty is just to the babies in their care. The midwives on postpartum wards also, understandably, believe their duty is to the women who actually have babies and are there on the ward. As a result, the women who don't have babies actually with them are left in a strange void in the middle, without help from either side. This is not anyone's fault as the staff are all working very hard with the patients they have, but it is a challenge when you're stuck in the middle and all you want is to see your baby. And don't get me started on actually getting pain relief. The drugs round is easily missed when you're sitting in NICU staring at your poorly offspring, and there's no way to get hold of anything in between times. After 24 hours of continuously missing the fabled trolley I asked John to bring me some paracetamol from home to take the edge off.

In total Ben spent a week in NICU. On the second day, his CRP (infection) levels went up and at 4:30am the NICU consultant came to me on the post-natal ward to get permission to perform a lumbar puncture to rule out meningitis. (All was fine, it was just a precaution and a short cause of IV antibiotics cleared the minor infection he'd contracted right up.) Naturally I gave immediate consent, although the consultant was a little startled I didn't require any further information before giving this. I was keen to hurry her out to get on with it – the sooner it was done the sooner any treatment could begin! I then spent a stressful and sleepless morning awaiting the results. In the middle of this, during the morning, a midwife came to see me to ask for a sputum sample. I was a bit confused, as was she, but apparently a message had been received by the midwives at the maternity unit from my CF hospital. My CF doctors were asking for the sample as I had grown a new bug in my last sputum sample, and they needed more of it to properly identify what bug it was. She was a little confused about the details of both the need for a sample and what my condition was, and we had a brief friendly chat about exactly what cystic fibrosis is, including why a sample was needed.

Needing to explain CF to medical professionals is surprisingly, and disturbingly, quite common. My GP at university was the worst – "CF? Remind me what that is again?" He asked me at the start of my signup appointment. I tried to jog his memory by saying it was the genetic disease that affected the lungs and pancreas, but he still looked blank. I hazarded "Faulty CFTR protein?", but he remained nonplussed, eventually declaring: "well! We'll have to learn about this one together, won't we!" It's sufficive to say that we did not. Usually non-CF specialist staff just have a momentary lapse and ask me how long I've had it, although I did once have a slightly heated row with a gynae nurse who swore blind that it was "not possible to catch cystic fibrosis in the vagina". To be fair she was technically correct, but it ended up being a very uncomfortable appointment for all the wrong reasons.

The midwife had no means of collecting a sample, so eventually I just coughed into a urine sample pot and she left, telling me that my CF sounded so horrible and time consuming, that must be why I was in my own room. I'd been moved out of a bay probably for that reason, as infection risks are naturally higher in hospitals, but I had slightly hoped it was the head midwife realising how horrible being baby-less on a ward full of babies is. Although the midwife had been nice, her parting comments left me feeling a little judged and suddenly uncertain that having a baby was a good idea.

Although common sense told me to be grateful that my CF team cared enough about my health that they had tracked me down to a maternity hospital less than 36 hours after I'd given birth to get hold of yet more lung gunk, my overwhelming feeling was one of frustration and sadness. I had just begun a whole new chapter in my life, brimming with potential and new experiences, but my CF had come with me, shattering the joy before I'd even had chance to hold my new baby properly. As I was just sat waiting for news I sank into a dark mood, depressed at how my baby could be so sick, and yet all I was doing was just worrying about my own wretched health, and whether I'd just made a huge mistake.

Fortunately, Ben did not have meningitis, he was weaned off oxygen and we went home as a little family seven days exactly after his birth. But I struggled to shift the uneasy feeling that brief post-partum conversation about CF had given me. The midwife had said nothing wrong, but I still felt a sense that she disapproved of me having a baby when my own health (as she perceived it) was poor. I began to worry about the things that I wouldn't live to see Ben do, and the different life experiences I would have to give him. Although I can see retrospectively it was just baby blues, it was a tough entry into motherhood.

-7-

DOUBLE TROUBLE

Having been warned by my doctors, and every other parent we'd met during my pregnancy, that having a baby would be a huge upheaval that would leave me exhausted and potentially cause my health to suffer, I was pleasantly surprised by how easy Ben was as a baby. He was always happy, always relaxed and even began to sleep through the night at a mere 10 weeks, much to the disgust of many of my other mum friends. By 9 months, John and I had reached a dangerous point in any parent's life. We became complacent, and decided that we were ready to start thinking about giving our son a sibling. Aware that I had actually been incredibly lucky with Ben, we agreed that I would speak to my doctor at my next clinic appointment to gauge their reaction and hear their thoughts on the idea.

Although we had good intentions, youthfulness, or perhaps carelessness, prevailed. Very soon after our conversation I realised that something had changed and that I was in fact already pregnant. We were surprised but happy, and I was guiltily glad that I didn't have to consult anyone as secretly common sense told me any doctor would tell me to wait and see how I got on with just one for at least a bit longer. We informed my CF team who congratulated us, and all seemed well. The only slight health hiccup was that my weight had not yet returned to my pre-pregnancy weight with Ben, something the doctors and dietitians were keen to get a hold on immediately.

Outside of the medical considerations, we were also in the process of John changing his job from an employed plumber working for a large company to becoming a self-employed one-man band. With our slightly unexpected news, we sat down and recalculated our figures. A brand-new business with two small children would be tricky, but it was doable. We knew it would be hard work, and certainly deeply stressful, but we felt that the long-term gain would be worth the short-term difficulties and so pressed on with finding a van, paying for a few additional qualifications and all the rigmarole that comes with setting up any new enterprise. At about week 6 of my pregnancy, I began to feel strange. I'd already had one pregnancy, so I knew what I was looking out for, but even so I was sure it was too early to be feeling the flutterings of a baby, yet I was certain I could. My womb felt like it was already stretching, and I was certain

I could feel the tiny little movements of a baby. At my 8 week check I mentioned this to my midwife, but she brushed it aside as being in my head. It hadn't been that long since my last pregnancy, so I'd remember the feeling, but I couldn't possibly already be feeling the baby move. By 9 weeks I succumbed to horrendous morning sickness. I was unable to do anything, and even drinking water made me vomit. After 7 days of constant sickness my weight was dropping and I visited the GP to ask for help. Again, my concerns about the pregnancy were brushed aside, and my GP simply gave me some dioralyte and told me not to worry. By my 12-week scan things were getting better, but I still felt an overwhelming feeling that something was different, and therefore wrong. On the Friday before my scan John finally handed in his four-week notice.

The scan was at 9 am on the Monday morning, and we drove through rush hour to the hospital. I had cautioned John that I felt something was wrong with the pregnancy, and we drove in silence, certain that the scan would show something awful. We sat in yet more silence in the waiting room, before nervously walking into the sonographer's room. The sonographer said hello and introduced us to the student who would be scanning me, her first experience on an actual patient. John sat close to the small screen, nervously chewing his fingers and we waited as the student carefully applied the gel. Being new, it took her a few minutes to locate the baby, which only fuelled the tension, but when she did it was instantly clear why I'd felt so ill. Two tiny babies swam on the screen, one even waving a miniature hand in a nonchalant, slightly mocking way. I gasped and looked at the student. She smiled at me, and it was obvious from my face that I knew what I was seeing, so she didn't verbalise what we were looking at on the screen. Unfortunately for John, he hadn't got the same level of scan experience as me. By this point I'd had 8 ultrasounds for my pregnancy with Ben, and on top of that have had an annual ultrasound from the age of four of my liver, kidneys and pancreas. Although this is not the same as looking at a baby, I always like to see what's going on and ask questions during my scans, and am getting reasonably good at deciphering the black and white, slightly speckled scan images as they appear on the screen. As a result, it took me no time at all to spot both the babies, see their movements and note that both hearts were beating well. John, who had to that point only seen two ultrasounds before in his whole life, was staring straight at the baby he could see at the centre of the screen, and was trying desperately to see if he could find the heart. He glanced up only briefly when the sonographer stood up and swapped places with the student – scanning twins thoroughly in the allocated appointment time is too much to ask a student on their first real life experience - and instead continued to study the little baby. The sonographer moved the probe over my belly, then calmly and matter-of-factly commented "all looks well. We have two heads, two hearts..." she stopped abruptly as John jumped back and fell off his chair. "TWO HEADS?? What??" Then he looked back at the screen, seeing the full picture for the first time. "You're joking. Its TWINS??" His face was a picture, and I couldn't help but laugh. It started out normally enough, but turned to a slightly hysterical and unstoppable giggle. I giggled with stress for the entire remainder of the appointment, apologising between outbursts. The sonographer was lovely and told me it was normal for mothers of multiples to react in odd ways upon discovering the news. Indeed, when we went to the reception to book in the next of many, many scans, the receptionist took one look at me giggling and John nervously pacing, then knowingly said "which is it then? Twins or triplets?" Whilst I laughed, John, at the opposite extreme, face already white as a sheet, turned slightly green at the mere mention of a third. Although the babies were looking good and healthy for 12-and-a-bit-weeks, the sonographer explained that they were MCDA twins, which meant they were sharing a placenta, but fortunately had separate amniotic sacs. This came with a range of potential problems, and we saw a consultant the next week who explained everything to us. The sonographer congratulated us warmly at the end of the appointment and asked if they would be our first. On learning we would be celebrating our son's first birthday at the end of that same week, she sucked breath in through her teeth and wished us luck.

My pregnancy with Ben did nothing to prepare me for carrying twins. Twin pregnancies are no joke, and I struggled for most of the 8 months. I am a tall but very slight woman, and the weight of two babies was hard to carry from very early on. Until I became pregnant with twins, I did not realise that all babies grow at the same rate for the first 20 weeks, no matter how many there are in the womb. This is because all organs need a certain amount of space to develop. There is a small range of sizes, but all healthy babies have to be within the range. This is how dating scans can be so accurate – the sonographers know exactly what measurements they're looking for. As a result, both my twins were growing quickly, and by 20 weeks their combined size and weight was equivalent to 32 weeks with Ben. My stomach muscles, built up by years of exercise and coughing, had stayed tight during my first pregnancy, and weren't showing any signs of giving in to the twins either. The babies were instead pushing up inside me, crushing my organs from the beginning. My bump appeared early on, but stayed small all the way through. Friends commented on its size, at first complementing its neatness, then openly telling me it was too small, it couldn't be that heavy, and how lucky I was to have another easy pregnancy. Strangers also passed judgement on it, with many a person questioning whether I was correct about it being twins. Yes. Yes, I know for a fact there are two, I said on repeat. I'm having more scans and appointments than I could ever possibly want, and they're both dancing on my bladder as we speak.

As well as the exhaustion of physically growing two babies whilst also taking care of another baby, I was also traipsing back and forth from hospital appointment to hospital appointment. My twins were sharing a placenta, which means that there was a high chance that at some point one of them would start hogging the nutrients and oxygen I was passing through it to them. This is called Twin-To-Twin-Transfusion Syndrome (TTTS), and is a dangerous and potentially fatal condition for both foetuses. To monitor this, as well as keep an eye on my CF and anticipated diabetes (although again, unbelievably, I did not get diabetes) the obstetrician saw me every two weeks. I had a scan as a part of these appointments to make sure that the babies were both growing well and evenly. Not to be outdone, my CF team decided to see me every other week as well. This was to keep a track of my weight (which was still far too low) and monitor my lung function. They were concerned that I was putting too much strain on myself, and wanted to be ahead of any potential exacerbations before they happened. Actually, this was never a problem, but I'm glad that they took so much care. This extra effort from two teams of physicians caused me to feel deeply irritated every time a friend commented how "easy" it was all going. I was pleased it was going well, but was very aware of how treacherous the situation was, and how little room there was for error.

By 29 weeks I was exhausted. The babies were never both asleep, and seemed to take it in turns to kick me all day and all night. Ben, having been an angelic small baby, teethed with a vengeance throughout my whole pregnancy. The poor boy did not teeth well, and actually cut all bar one tooth more than once, as they kept appearing and then disappearing back into his gums, almost taunting us that we would be double teething again with our next babies. When he finally cut his last tooth, aged nearly three, I almost cried with relief, the experience had been so harrowing. Not that the girls have been much better. They average 3 sleepless screaming nights and days for each tooth, and follow each other exactly, which results in 6 nights of lost sleep and much frustrated shouting for every blinking tooth. To make matters worse Freya has actually cut a supernumerary (extra) tooth in the roof of her mouth as well, which took a staggering 8 days to come through, as if we didn't have enough of the things to deal with already.

On top of teething, Ben also refused to walk until he was nearly 16 months old, almost as though he sensed this was his last chance to be constantly cuddled by me. I therefore spent most of my pregnancy carrying a very heavy weight everywhere, Ben being a particularly large and hefty baby. Eventually, at 7 months pregnant,

I refused to carry him anymore. I couldn't do it, he was physically too heavy for me and squashed my already uncomfortable bump every time I tried. After crying about it for less than ten minutes he got up and wandered off, remarkably steady on his feet for a child taking his first steps. Rather than celebrating his "first steps", I was infuriated by them, and wondered how long the monster had been keeping his mobility a secret.

At 30 weeks John and I took a trip to Ikea with his parents to buy cots and other necessities for our new arrivals. As we get out of the car I became aware of a large amount of liquid running down my legs, soaking my maternity leggings. We sat in the café, waiting to see if I was about to go into labour, but nothing happened. John's parents were sympathetic, repeatedly telling me not to worry, pregnant women lose control of their bladders all the time. The next day I went for yet another scan, and the sonographer discovered that the amniotic sac around the lower twin was all but empty of fluid. This was a potential sign of TTTS, although the twins were still very close in size. The obstetrician decided the best course of action was to start having weekly scans, and told me to keep my hospital bag packed and in the car ready. When I got home I told John this, and he stressed about the possibility of the twins having problems and needing to be born too early. Although I was concerned about this, I was more interested in having him get on the phone to his parents and inform them I didn't wet myself in an Ikea car park.

Fortunately the sac refilled, and although the twins stopped growing at this point, neither stole from the other, and the pregnancy continued to limp on. In essence, they simply ran out of room. There was no more space in my body for them to grow into, and they stayed small from that point forwards. For the final 6 weeks I cried every night, I was so hormonal, so exhausted but unable to sleep. John didn't know what to do, opting to keep his head down, regularly bringing me a Calshake with a slightly sheepish expression on his face. Ben started to have nightmares and I spent a disproportionate number of the remaining nights walking up and down the landing, rocking a large toddler in my arms. After yet another CF appointment, my consultant's letter to my GP said I was "visibly tired". I'm pretty sure this was a polite way of saying "she looks like crap", and I had to concur with his observation. Eventually my obstetrician took pity on me, and at my 35+6 week scan she decided to call time, asking me to come in the next morning for induction. I was so relieved I almost kissed her, and headed home delighted that it was almost over.

After a long, sleepless night we arrived at the hospital for 9am sharp, all happy and ready to go. I felt like I knew the drill – it had only been 17 months since my last baby. This time I was taken straight to the delivery ward. MCDA twins are extremely high risk, and my previous labour had been on the fast side. I was admitted, and they began to monitor the babies. As always, they struggled to find both heart beats – twin one was always tricky and so what should have been an hour quickly became two. Finally, they had all the things they needed and moved on to explain the induction process. This wasn't new to me and I politely nodded along.

Three hours later our midwife popped her head round the door. "We're just a bit busy I'm afraid love, so sit tight." Lunch came. We continued to wait. At approximately 9pm the head midwife for the new shift arrived and explained, in a rather strained voice, that they were very busy, and in fact they were closing the unit. They didn't want to send me home in case anything changed (I was now 36 weeks with placenta sharing twins and they were hoping they could start induction sooner rather than later) so John went home alone.

The next morning we waited again. Again I was monitored – this now took 2 and a half hours as twin 1 was such a fidget – but again we had to wait. There was another lovely midwife, another bizarre lunch and then the news came – we could begin. My midwife went to get the necessary prescription.

Two hours later she returned and apologetically told me the lady next door was "having trouble" and they would wait for her baby to be born before they induced me in case her baby required one of our NICU cots.

John and I went for a short walk, although for me this felt like a waddle, before struggling to get back into the delivery unit as the buzzer wasn't being answered. At last a doctor turned up behind us and opened the door to go in. He looked at both of us. "Who are you visiting?" he asked suspiciously. Somewhat frustrated I replied "it's me. And it's twins. We're room 12." Slightly embarrassed the poor man let us in and raced off. I should probably have been grateful he hadn't thought I looked like a whale, but I found the size of my bump to be awkward. At 8 months with twins most other women guessed about 5 months with one.

Lo and behold, on our way back down the DU corridor we passed the unfortunate baby being raced by our midwife and a team of doctors off to the NICU. She smiled apologetically at me, her focus flicking straight back to the silent baby in the cot. Somewhat deflated we went and sat back in room 12. As predicted a few hours later our midwife arrived to confirm that no, my induction would not be taking place that afternoon.

That evening shift changes happened and a bubbly student midwife came into our room. "I've come to monitor the babies ready to start your induction!" she grinned. My heart sank slightly. Normally, I love a student. They need to learn and I'll always allow a student take blood or examine me or even just sit in, and can never understand people who don't. After all, if no one ever lets anyone but the most experienced clinician treat them how will anyone learn? Better to let a student have a go when they are supervised, thus allowing knowledge to be passed down so that everyone can improve. In all honesty students can often be better at things such as taking blood than their more experienced colleagues. Yes, there is a risk they might have to do it twice, but they always seem to be gentler about it. The more experienced the nurse the more accurate, yet more brutal, they seem to be. That being said, I'm not new to the hospital world and I knew instantly that a student on her own was not about to begin the induction for such a high-risk case. Still we chatted on and I reassured her it was ok that she couldn't find twin one – "no one ever can!" and finally we had done all the monitoring and tests. She took the results off to the main midwife and returned with the predicted news. No NICU space, so no babies tonight. Frustrated I requested that I be allowed to go home for the night. The flustered student got the head midwife and we agreed that as I'd been sat around for 36 hours, a night in my own bed would be good. So long as I checked back in at 9 am the next morning.

At 9 am the next morning I was informed that there were still no NICU cots. Perturbed I inquired what would happen if I just went in to labour (by now I had lost the mucus plug, which is a sign of imminent labour, and had twice over the preceding few weeks been in the hospital with contractions.) The midwife shuffled nervously and informed me that if they came and there

141

was a problem the babies would be blue lighted to other units. And so I sat tight and we continued to wait.

I went home again that night, still wearing my hospital bands and my allergy band. The staff were all very apologetic, and very grateful to me and John that we hadn't kicked up a fuss. Every time a staff member came in they looked increasingly nervous, bracing themselves for the torrent of abuse they thought we would throw at them. We reassured them we understood why, and appreciated that they had the babies' best interests at heart. What we didn't say was that we had now spent 3 whole days sitting on a delivery unit, with babies being born literally all round us. Those walls are not as thick as you'd think. Despite this I was actually angered to see that the staff were just presuming we would shout at them. As a heavy user of the NHS, I cannot understand anyone who gets angry when they're waiting for treatment. For a start, it's free. FREE. And secondly, if you are waiting in a hospital it is because you aren't top priority, which means you are not dying. BE GRATEFUL. As I was soon to find out, if one does suddenly have a near death experience the staff will be with you quicker than you can say "is this normal?" Politeness and kindness cost nothing, so just let everyone do their jobs. No-one wants to hurt you in a hospital, they want to help you. Apart from phlebotomists, but they can't help it.

We began day four with a less than perfect start. My room on the delivery unit had been given to a more needing person, AKA: a woman who was actually in labour, and therefore my daily twin monitoring began in a separate clinic. This was a special outpatient clinic, where women with little worries were sent to be reassured. I had been here several times over both pregnancies already. Again, monitoring took an age, but this time I received a visit at the end from a consultant and a registrar. We were informed that today was the last day, and babies needed to come. If there weren't enough NICU cots in an hour's time I would be sent on my way. Possibly to Liverpool, possibly to London. They were a bit hazy on where, but I was definitely going. Somewhat nervously I was moved to a recently vacated room on the delivery unit. It smelt very clean, and I (slightly selfishly) hoped all had gone fantastically.

Another doctor, Doctor Sam, visited me with his two brand-new medical students and passed the time by demonstrating a complete maternal exam for the students and then having them do one each for practice. This sounds a strange way to spend an hour, but I'm always happy to help with teaching new doctors and quite enjoy learning new things that I'll never need to know or use again. As a teenager, I once had a severe reaction to a substance I spilt in a biology lesson at school and spent several days in the hospital. The highlight of these days was having the consultant regularly shove students and juniors in to my room to diagnose me. "Ignore all the facial swelling, and the nasty rash. They're a red herring. Just find out what's really wrong with her." They never got it, and the consultant would come back later to high five me for being such a tricky patient.

Suddenly, we were ready. Cots were there and had been fully reserved. I was slightly dubious they could keep NICU cots for unborn babies, but I later met the head NICU nurse, and understood how this could be possible. She was not a lady to be crossed. Excited to finally meet the babies I was slightly discouraged when we were moved off Delivery Unit to the adjacent ward, and then further discouraged when they sent John off to get dinner for himself. Unsure what was happening I paced the ward for a member of staff. "I'm supposed to be being induced, am I at the right place? Are you sure? Not delivery unit?" I could tell the poor midwife felt I was harassing her, but by this time I'd spent four whole days there and was not about to get lost in the system. Sounding exasperated, she convinced me to go back to my bed and jabbed me with a steroid injection for good measure.

After what felt like an age, a stressed and tetchy John finally returned. Maternity units are like Fort Knox for the Dads. If they're not with a large, preferably screaming, woman then they will just be left to stand outside for hours whilst staff rush around inside, too busy to push the door open button. Bizarrely they are often watched by the dads who have gotten inside but daren't press the button for fear of incurring the wrath of the over stressed midwife. Not too much more time passed, and we were escorted by our latest midwife back to the delivery unit. At last we were underway. At 6pm she finally put in the gel and said, "we'll just try this for now, but I'll leave a note for the next shift and they can give you a stronger dose if there's nothing happening in 6 hours." How little did we know.

Now that I had finally begun the induction process I was keen to get off the delivery unit and have a stroll to stretch my legs. I'd been too nervous before in case I missed my chance, but now I was raring to go. We casually wandered out of the unit and into the corridor. Already I could feel the strange tightening effect of the gel. We wandered along, our gait getting quicker and quicker as the tightening became stronger. After about 50 minutes I called time and we headed swiftly back to the unit. I knew things were about to get started. At two minutes to 7 I went to the loo for a quick wee. A surprisingly large amount of blood appeared in the water, so John called the midwife. She appeared quickly, but without too much concern she told me to just lie down whilst she fetched a doctor. She didn't think it was too much blood and the water was probably making it seem worse. As she left I felt my first contraction. It was agonising and accompanied by a huge gush of blood.

John called the midwife down the corridor, who rushed back. She took one look, casually pulled the giant red panic! button and said "oh, that's quite a lot of blood there" with such composure she could easily have been commenting on a new nail varnish colour, not the Niagara Falls of blood that was pouring out of me. Within seconds the room was absolutely full. There were doctors, midwives, anaesthetists, students. It was a big room, and I had been pre-warned by my obstetrician that as I was an unusual case every man and his dog would want to watch, but even in the throes of incredibly fierce contractions I couldn't believe the sheer number of bodies.

Without any ado, the physicians jumped into action. Two anaesthetists began putting cannulas in, one on each side of me. Doctor Sam was ultra-sounding the babies to establish heart rates, another doctor was asking questions, the midwife was giving me gas and air and two others were simultaneously undressing me and putting a gown on. This sounds chaotic, but they were so calm and in tune it felt like I was part of a strangely choreographed dance. The doctors began to explain in very fast voices that they were taking me for an emergency caesarean section, pausing uncertainly when the contractions were too strong for me to keep my eyes open. I told them I was still listening – I'm no fool and could tell from both the rate that blood was making an exit, and the speed of their voices, that without much haste this was not going to end well. They whizzed me across the corridor at speed to the handily adjacent operating theatre (I found out later they had been partially expecting this sort of scenario, given the size of my double placenta and precipitous nature of my previous labour, and had therefore planned accordingly) where one of the anaesthetists began calmly, yet somehow frantically, to administer a spinal block. By this point the contractions had melded together to be just one agonising pain, and the midwives held me still so she could get the needle into my spine as safely as possible. I then laid down and she tilted the table so my head was considerably lower than my feet and started throwing ice at me to see if I could still feel my legs. By this time, I was very aware that the blood loss was already huge and still ongoing, and I was quietly beginning to panic. The staff all looked calm, but I felt that doctors covered in blood before a c-section had even begun was not a good sign. Time seemed to stand still as everyone in the room just watched and waited for the spinal to kick in, eyes flicking from me to the clock on the wall and back. John was stood just to my left, looking terrified, with a midwife next to him. I wasn't sure when, but he'd changed into dark blue scrubs, and someone had shoved a surgical hat on his head. It sat crookedly, the scrubs were far too large and he looked ridiculously out of place amongst the professionals. Meanwhile a somewhat startled sounding midwife was calling "4, 5, 6..." to the crowd. This confused me until the doctor took over with a surprised "10! Wow! Ok, let's do this naturally then!"

It had taken me less than 10 minutes to reach 10 centimetres dilation. They returned the bed to a horizontal position, just as the spinal finally kicked in and, after quickly confirming that both babies were still doing well, they informed me they were going to use forceps "just in case" and it was all systems go.

Freya came out first, quickly and easily. Her face had been squashed by months of her sister sitting on it, but she was fine. She was briefly shown to me and John, the doctor kindly taking a second to ask John what the sex was, knowing we'd deliberately chosen to have a surprise. "IT'S A GIRL!" he shouted, a combination of relief, adrenaline and sheer panic escaping all at once. I was delighted. We had opted not to find out the sex, but somehow convinced ourselves we were having two more boys, and we were shocked and ecstatic in equal measure. Then she was whisked off to the paediatricians, and I was told to start pushing again. Twin 2 was breech, they said, but there was not enough time to try and turn her. Eve came quickly enough, and again we were quickly shown her before she vanished off. The doctors speedily helped the placenta out, Doctor Sam using what looked like his entire bodyweight to push down on my stomach whilst the other doctor pulled. My placenta, I was told later, had come away almost entirely from my womb wall with the sheer force of the contractions, and I was haemorrhaging blood terribly as a result. In order to stop this the placenta needed to be completely removed so my body would naturally stop bleeding. The doctors managed this very quickly, checked it over to make sure it was all in one piece, then both breathed an audible sigh of relief. Freya and Eve, weighing 3lb 14oz and 4lb 4oz, had both been born safely within 23 minutes of my labour starting. After a four day wait for induction to begin the speed of their arrival had definitely taken us all by surprise.

With a palpable sense of relief, the observing doctors, midwives, paediatricians and anaesthetists all began offering their congratulations before quickly disappearing off to save lives and welcome new arrivals. The remaining staff washed the blood off me, and things turned slightly comical as four of them; the two delivering doctors and two midwives, braced themselves and then transferred me swiftly from the operating table to a waiting hospital bed as I was effectively paralysed from just above my waist down to my toes. I'm not a heavy woman, and they hadn't adjusted their efforts for my tiny frame, instead catapulting me from one bed to the other, almost throwing me off onto the floor. Doctor Sam swore out loud, catching me at the last second, all professionalism gone. They all laughed, joking that I was probably the lightest just post-partum mother they'd ever had, but breaking my hip after they'd just gotten me through such a traumatic childbirth would probably reflect poorly on them, all extremely jovial now that the crisis was over. The doctors left, and the midwives pushed me round to the Close Observation Unit. By now

I was feeling very cold and shaking uncontrollably, but the nurse I was handed over too reassured me this was just the spinal block and the shock of how fast everything had progressed. She took my SATs and BP, whilst chatting to me about her niece. A new addition to the family, the poor girl had been born with cystic fibrosis. I offered my condolences and we proceeded to chat about the advancements in care that were taking place and which forms of exercise I considered most helpful as an aid for physio.

Out of nowhere I suddenly felt an all-consuming chill and fear run through me. I looked at John, who had by this point been allowed back in. I didn't realise it at the time, but he told me later that the second Eve was born he was swiftly removed from the theatre by a very stern midwife whilst the doctors worked on stopping me from bleeding out. I turned to him, said, "I don't feel very well." Before promptly dropping backwards onto my pillow, the room spinning in and out of focus. Although hazy, I can vaguely picture another large team of physicians standing over me, and was aware of a lot of voices calling my name, instructions to each other and a variety of numbers. Someone was taking my pulse, someone else my temperature. A nurse started pushing a clear liquid through a syringe into the veins on the back of my hand, whilst a doctor had attached a bag of blood to a cannula located at my elbow and was squeezing it to speed up its flow. On the other side, an anaesthetist introduced himself to me and explained he was putting in an arterial line. Slightly giddy, I told him my veins were sometimes a bit tricky, so it might take him a while. The man was a true professional and smiled through my condescending comment, easily accessing my artery and sewing the line in to allow continuous blood pressure checks. Someone else put an oxygen mask over my face. My new, somewhat flustered, consultant (the twins were born at a shift change, which explains why the operating theatre had been SO full) ran about ordering a chest x-ray and frantically calling for more blood, whilst also phoning intensive care to see if they could take me. Someone else tucked the bed clothes right down, layered blankets on top and pushed what felt like a very large, very hot leaf blower under all the covers to try and raise my plummeting body temperature. I saw John being rather forcefully led away by a midwife, but I'm afraid the room went dark, and I remember nothing else.

-8-

LIFE WITH CHILDREN

I awoke in a panic at about 2 am. John was asleep in a chair by my side, and I still had oxygen prongs in my nose. I called to him, confused and concerned that the hospital might not know we were still there. What if something happened to the girls? They might phone our home and we'd miss it. John reassured me it was ok, the staff definitely knew where we were, and the lovely nurse organised for Eve to be brought down from the NICU for a cuddle to ease my worries. I held her tiny frame in my arms and went back to sleep, this time in a peaceful haze.

When I awoke early the next morning my oxygen was gone, and I felt fit and raring to go. The nurse, seeing I was awake, sent John off to get himself some breakfast. Slightly concerned I asked the nurse if the spinal was still working, as I couldn't feel anything. Concerned, she started slapping my legs, much harder than her slim arms suggested she would be able to. I stopped her very quickly – I had merely meant I could feel no pain. This was not my first natural birth experience, and I was well aware of the post-partum pain I should be feeling, even without such a traumatic experience. Surprised, the nurse shushed me "everyone on this unit has had a bad c-section or birth experience, so don't say that out loud!" she whispered. I had, thanks to the skill of the doctors, come through a traumatic forceps and breech forceps birth with no stitches and minimal bruising. Chuffed with this, I requested that I be allowed to go to the bathroom on my own. This was allowed, my catheter was removed, and I was soon dressed and waiting for the doctor to visit.

The consultant, somewhat taken aback to find me fully clothed and sitting in the chair next to the bed, less than 13 hours after a somewhat traumatic birth, told me she'd come to check on me ahead of ward round to be certain I was ok. She wanted to make sure I understood what had happened so I wouldn't be shocked when one of her juniors presented my case. She explained that I had received three units of blood due to a placental abruption and subsequent haemorrhage, but she was very pleased with the progress of my recovery. She informed me they believed I had lost around 2.1 litres of blood, and as a result had gone into hypovolemic shock, specifically hemorrhagic shock. A person cannot survive losing more than 2.2 litres, and I was therefore lucky to be alive. Although chilling, the fact that I was alive and it was all over with no harm done was really all I took from her comments and therefore politely declined her offer to sign me up for a course of counselling. The babies were doing well, although they needed tube feeding for weight gain, and I was looking forward to leaving this episode behind me and moving forwards as a family of five.

Before the end of the day I was transferred to the normal post-partum ward. I was back in the same side room I'd been in only 17 months before, once again the baby-less mother on a ward filled with screaming babies. This time I was more mentally prepared, and embraced the last few days of peace and relatively uninterrupted sleep. The girls were moved out of NICU and onto the Special Care Baby Unit (SCBU) as their only requirement was tube feeding. I went to visit them with John, but the nurses told me to take it easy and use the opportunity to sleep. They'd been following our progress since we first arrived for induction five days ago, my name having popped up again and again on the board, waiting for the cots, and one of them told me she'd managed to sneak across and see my labour. I was slightly disturbed by this, childbirth not being the most dignified of situations, but I took her advice and went back to bed. In the corridor leading down to the ward a doctor called out my name. She raced up and congratulated me, expressing her delight that I was so well recovered as I'd looked "horrendous" last night. She was smartly dressed and well turned out, and I'm embarrassed to admit I didn't immediately recognise her. Then I pinpointed her voice and realised she was the other blood covered, scrubs wearing doctor pulling twins out of me a mere 18 hours previously. I thanked her profusely for her hard work and fast actions and she disappeared off deeper into the hospital, proclaiming that seeing a quick recovery like mine made her job feel fantastic.

After a further day, the doctors decided that I could go home, and at 11am they set about discharging me. Having experienced enough hospital discharges to know that this is not a quick task, I headed off to the SCBU and spend a good few hours cuddling my babies. At about 4pm I checked in at the ward to see if there'd been any progress. The midwives were all busy, but the clerk informed me that they were still waiting on pharmacy; my large blood loss had led the doctor to prescribe iron tablets. Unperturbed I left again, unsurprised that there was a wait on drugs. By 8pm, however, I started to get a little impatient that there'd been no progress. The clerk had long gone and the midwives told me I'd just have to wait and go in the morning. John, who had been sitting with me for an hour or so whilst his mother walked 17-month-old Ben up and down the corridor, headed home, telling me to call him when I needed a lift. The next morning I got up, saw the girls and waited. By midday, I was getting annoyed. I sought out the ward clerk, who was looking stressed, and enquired how my discharge was going. I was not on her list, and she asked what time I was told I could go home. When I said 11 o'clock she snorted in derision and told me there was no way I could expect to be done in an hour. When I informed her that it had in fact been 25, she was taken aback and started to look through the previous days notes. We were apparently still waiting on pharmacy, and I wandered back to SCBU. By that night, I was cheesed off. The ward clerk had again left, and it was up to a midwife to tell me I was going to have to stay in. I contemplated self-discharge, but the midwife told me the iron tablets were very important, so I stayed. As I was in the discharge pile I hadn't actually had any iron tablets for two days by that point, but that didn't cross my mind until after she'd already gone. The next morning the midwives turfed me out of the side room into a bay as, despite technically being an infection risk, they felt I was taking up too much space. I sat in the bay, watching the woman in my room cuddling her own new born twins, seething with jealousy. The woman looked relaxed, baby clutched in her arms, her husband happily holding the other whilst simultaneously holding his wife's hand. After a while he spotted me staring, got up and closed the curtain. My twins, meanwhile, were in SCBU and I was too nervous about missing the elusive pharmacy delivery to go and see them. The other women in the bay were all also waiting for discharge. They all had a bump, a baby, a waiting husband, a car seat and a large amount of baggage. They chatted amongst themselves, comparing notes on labour and complaining about how long discharge takes – one of them had been waiting 6 hours! The horror! I didn't join in, and they didn't invite me to. To be honest I looked both irritable and like I'd slipped in under false pretences. I'd already sent my hospital bag home (under the false assumption I would be following it quicker than I did) John was in the SCBU, and I was back in jeans as my maternity trousers refused to stay up as my bump had vanished almost the second I'd given birth. The only item I had was a book, which I tried to read. Only an amateur attends a hospital without a book. At 1 o'clock, a whole 50 hours after the doctor first said I could go home, the midwives arrived to tell me I could finally leave. There were four of them at the entrance to the bay, and they were all carrying a box of medication. It turned out that a slight mix up meant that the midwives (or perhaps the doctor) had prescribed a month's supply of all of my CF meds, including supplements, not just a two-week supply of iron tablets, and they'd had to order them in. The other women all broke off from their moaning and stared open-mouthed at me, clearly wondering what could possibly have gone wrong in my labour that I needed this many drugs. John came back from the SCBU, rolled his eyes, and we tried to leave with dignity, eight days since first arriving for induction, both of us hauling two large boxes through the unit and out to the car.

After a bit of back and forwards to the maternity hospital, and then our more local hospital to see the girls in the SCBU, they were finally discharged 13 days after their speedy birth. We thanked the staff at the hospital, bundled our still tiny daughters into their ridiculously large looking car seats and attempted to make a swift journey home. This proved harder than we thought. Leaving a small hospital on a Saturday lunchtime with two infant car seats and a small toddler caused something of a stir. The hospital wasn't as bustling as usual, and we were a painfully obtrusive family. John was balancing spare blankets and a car seat with a 4lb baby in on one arm whilst tightly gripping the hand of a bemused, slightly reluctant 17-month-old with the other hand. I was struggling with the other car seat with another 4lb baby in and all their bottles and baby clothes just behind. In the corridor patients smiled and cooed. As we walked through the shop and café area towards the exit visitors and outpatients called "Double trouble!" and "good luck!" Slightly surprised, but caught in an adrenaline bubble of finally leaving the hospital we smiled and thanked people. When we got to the door we realised it was raining, so John ran off to get the car whilst I bent down to put Ben's coat on. We'd put the car seats on the floor behind me, and within seconds I was swamped. Elderly women were bending down to admire the girls, guess their sexes and tell me whether or not they were identical. Someone else was complimenting me on getting my figure back so quickly, and another person was trying to tell me their daughter had just found out she was having twins. The voices all blurred together, and I started to get a little stressed by all the faces in my tiny, tiny babies faces. As I tried to pull both the car seats away from all these strangers Ben began to cry. It was a baptism of fire and a preparation for what was to come.

For some reason, a large number of people think it's ok to just stop anyone with multiples and ask all number of innocuous questions, sometimes photographing them at the same time. Questions are fine, although photos are not. I was happy to smile and chat with people at first, but soon a quick trip (ha! "quick" with three under two is impossible) to the supermarket was doubling in length as random strangers stopped to quiz me on everything from sleeping habits to birth weights, or simply to tell me they once knew someone who'd had twins. If I had a penny for every time someone has shouted, "Double trouble! You've got your hands full!" at me, I'd no longer have a mortgage. I don't mind too much, but some people can just be rude. The worst thing I've ever heard was a woman who bent down and asked if the girls were identical. I said they were, and she looked closely at them both, then declared they couldn't be as "that one's pretty." It's getting easier as the children are getting older, but the number of people who made bizarre remarks about my family planning situation in the early days was quite shocking.

There are some people who appear to believe it's possible to plan twins, and more than a few have stopped me and asked how they too can fall pregnant twice over. The honest answer is even if there was a way I really wouldn't advise it. I love my twins, but they are hard work. There's a reason most women pop out one at a time. Also, on behalf of all multiple parents everywhere, please can people stop announcing their children's age gap and claiming it's "basically the same as having twins." If your children's age gap is measured in months not minutes, it's just not the same. At all.

Life with three children under two can only be described as pure chaos. From day one we hit the ground running. John's business being in its infancy meant he couldn't take any more time off as paternity leave as we'd spent so much time hanging round the hospital waiting to be induced and then to be discharged. He actually went back to work a week before the girls were allowed home, and we had to delay them coming home from a Friday to a Saturday so he could be with me. This was met with disgust by our less than friendly new SCBU nurse, but needs must and with three children and a mortgage we didn't really have a choice. My mum started coming down every couple of weeks for a few days to help out, but even then it was madness. Every day was full of nappies, washing was endless and every week there were 60 little nails to cut after bath time. For reasons I'm not entirely sure of (probably denial at my own prolific fertility) I decided during my pregnancy that my current buggy could just have another seat attached, and I didn't need to buy a triple buggy. I reasoned, hormonally, that Ben was basically a small child, not a toddler, and wouldn't go in the buggy much anyway. At 17 months he'd been walking all of 8 weeks, so this was, in hindsight, a ridiculous idea. Instead I spent most of the following 18 months pushing a heavy double buggy, carrying either a twin in a sling or Ben on my back whilst also holding the dog lead with my other hand.

As the girls had come home weighing only 4lb and 4lb 1, I had been strictly instructed to feed them every three hours. I had lost so much weight breastfeeding Ben for 6 months that I didn't even attempt to feed the girls myself. This was undoubtedly for the best, especially with a toddler running around as well, but life appeared to be just one continuous bottle wash. The girls had terrible reflux, which we dealt with by winding for a good half hour after every feed. This worked well, but was deeply time consuming. I went to a twins group to see if I could meet other twin mums in a similar situation, but over time it became harder and harder to comfortably sit there and chat. Many of the other mothers were, understandably, suspicious of me. Most twins are small, premature and a lot have additional health problems. Since having my own twins, it's actually been my health that hasn't been brilliant, and the presence of a very skinny woman who won't stop coughing was clearly uncomfortable for a lot of them. On more than one occasion, a mother actually moved her tiny offsprings out of my vicinity, slightly tutting at me as she did. Initially I persevered anyway, and I did make a few friends, but I eventually stopped going to avoid the awkwardness.

In addition to both waking separately in the night for feeds, the girls were much more prone to illness than Ben ever was. In the run up to their first Christmas they both developed chesty coughs that kept them awake all day and night. We kept returning to our GP who was sympathetic and watched them carefully, even phoning us at 9pm on a Friday evening to check how they were doing, but they were always just well enough to not need any further care. After a couple of weeks of this we went in late to the GP for an emergency appointment before we headed up north to my parents for Christmas. The GP was unsure what to do with them, and decided to send us to the local hospital children's ward to be checked. The girls were monitored and we were discharged at 11pm. We went home, collected the dog, and drove on up to Manchester through the night. My parents suggested we might be better getting some sleep and waiting till the morning, but quite frankly with two-month-old twins and a 19-month-old we didn't know what the difference between day and night was, both being so sleep deprived they had blurred into one.

As well as the day to day chaos that is life with three little ones, I also have to factor in hospital time. Child care for three tiny children on an ad-hoc basis is often difficult to come by. This is a recurrent problem, as my hospital appointments are regular but not always at the same time. Therefore, I usually bring the whole gang with me. This was fine when it was just Ben, one baby being a huge bonus - something to play with for the few hours I sit around for. The staff all cooed over him, and unbelievably he never once even cried during an appointment. When the girls arrived it was a logistical challenge, but at first they were happy to sit in the buggy and look round. Now I have three toddlers, however, things have gotten tricky. Every month I think I can handle a couple of hours trapped in a room in clinic with them, always hopeful, and almost always dead wrong. I bring books, puzzles, toys and copious amounts of treats and snacks, and you'd be amazed how long tiny children can stretch hide and seek out in a room with only 2 chairs, a desk and a curtain. Despite all my efforts to entertain them however, at some point during all appointments the children begin to wreak havoc. They fight over their snacks, their toys and at one point during an appointment last year my son actually climbed up onto the couch in the corner and leapt off, caterwauling like a mini Tarzan. The doctor looked wary, but politely ignored the chaos. I was really trying to listen to what she was saying, but I kept having to break away to admonish my little Huns. I gave Ben a death stare, but as he was only two and a half he didn't pick up on the imminent peril he'd put himself in. It's a good job the doctor was there to be honest, as without a witness I'd probably have done something I'd have later regretted.

In fairness, although my children aren't exactly placid at the best of times, asking anyone to sit and wait in a hot room for a few hours to answer the same questions every month is a bit of a tall order. If I could get away with seeing how far I can jump from the couch in the corner I probably would. Clinic appointments are absolutely vital, but that doesn't make them exciting. That being said my children are learning a lot from being around hospitals so regularly. They spend a lot of time playing doctors, and I never know whether to be proud or disturbed when they take the syringe from the obligatory toy doctor's kit we have, carefully wipe the arm (or eyelid, face or foot) of their patient with a tissue, then stab at them to "take blood. I take blood."

Every now and again I will meet someone who is new to the CF team, and is therefore slightly surprised when they open the clinic room door to a nursery. When the new dietitian walked in for the first time she gasped and cried "aww look at all these! They're so sweet!" The children responded by staring open mouthed at her in a slightly menacing way. Wrong footed she backed away from them and sat down, turning her attention to me and asking, "Are they all yours then?" I paused briefly, wondering who would be crazy enough to bring three children under the age of three to a hospital appointment out of choice, without even a genetic link to them. Then I realised that the dietitian clearly thought I looked that mad, and with my slightly wild expression, odd socks and un-brushed hair, I really couldn't blame her.

Other than the odd person getting a shock, the staff seem to be very accepting of my rabble. Nevertheless, there is a definite split between those who have had children themselves and those who are blissfully ignorant of the pandemonium children cause. The former talk to me over the children, able to completely ignore what's going on around them, whilst the latter repeatedly break off mid-sentence, distracted by the wanton anarchy toddlers create. This attitude runs through more than just the actual appointment. All the staff are kind and tell me they know my life is probably a bit tricky at the moment, and how hard it must be to keep up with treatments, but there's a definite difference in the level of appreciation between the two camps. During one of my more recent appointments, a rare child free affair, the physiotherapist suggested more exercise would be beneficial for my lungs. Obviously she was completely correct, and she smiled at me politely as I said time might be an issue, innocently asking if it was all getting a bit easier now the children were all a bit older. I hesitated briefly, thinking back to an hour earlier. As I was going to the hospital where I would be seeing actual people I thought I should probably sneak in a quick shower, it having been approximately four days since I'd last accomplished that basic task. Midway through washing my hair one twin declared she'd pooed, and I needed to wipe her bottom. I stuck my head through the shower curtain to see she'd not only pooed and spread it everywhere, but her sister had opened and spilt a tub of wall paint all over the floor. She was currently stood in it, attempting to scrape it all back into the tub with her hands. I jumped out, unsure which disaster to tackle first, when Ben called up from downstairs that he'd opened the door and the dog had escaped. Fearing Ben would run out onto the road to get him back I raced downstairs and was almost out the door when John came up the drive, having finished early so I could have the luxury of an appointment on my own. He was somewhat surprised to see his soapy haired wife about to exit the house naked. It's a good job he was there really – we live in a very small, rather conservative village and I'm pretty certain we're already known as the loud family with too many children for our tiny house and a miscreant escaping dog. I'm not sure "streaker" is the best thing to add to the list. I didn't really know how to relate this not unusual story to the physiotherapist without potentially putting her off children for life, so I kept to the fight club rules of parenting and instead quietly muttered something about it being "just different, really."

In a category of their own sits the new parents. They are always delighted to see the children, and the children take full advantage of the situation. Once when I had to come to the day ward unexpectedly for a repeat lung function test and bloods after starting new antibiotics at a clinic appointment, I met such a staff member. I packed the children, Ben aged two and the girls aged one, into the car with the usual paraphernalia, and we headed to the hospital. Unfortunately, I didn't consider how long it would take to be seen by respiratory physiology (spirometry), a nurse and a doctor. Without children, this would have been a painless irritation, but with them it was a nightmare. I hadn't allowed for the fact that the day ward is long and thin, and the children would not be contained to a room. They realised this within seconds of getting there, running up and down in opposite directions like lunatics. I tried to control them, but as the girls were only 14 months this prooved impossible, and I ended up spending a good few hours running around after them, apologising to nurses and other patients with every other breath, especially when Ben lay down and stuck his head under a closed curtain to grin at the man in the bed behind. After I'd had my breathing tests a young doctor came down to see me, pulling the magical NHS soundproof curtain shut to give us some privacy. He then saw the children and grinned, telling me he had just had one of his own.

To me it seems that new parents are always keen to interact with toddlers, probably seeing them as an insight into their own future, hopefully one that has less overflowing nappies and fewer sleepless nights. Unfortunately, they don't realise (or I certainly didn't) that when their tiny bundle of joy becomes a chubby, adorable toddler then actually they will look back longingly to those early days when their little monster didn't run away, and crying was the result of a limited number of options not the irrational tantrum of a small child whose favourite cup is suddenly and inexplicably the wrong colour, or whose biscuit is just that bit too biscuity. They have no idea that in the future they will have lost all sense of what is acceptable behaviour to the point where they won't think twice to opening the door and accepting a neighbour's parcel whilst simult-aneously wiping their child's bottom behind the half open door with their other hand. The sense of hope and excitement around a new parent in the first few months before they realise just how much chaos they've wilfully introduced into their own life is almost tangible. This doctor was no different, and he immediately crouched down to say hello, delighted to meet three tiny toddlers.

Unfortunately, he picked my most melodramatic daughter to introduce himself to. As if she could sense the poor man's weakness, she launched herself backwards in a completely unnecessary display of faux fear, falling through the curtain and cracking her head on the metal table behind her. Instantly, blood exploded out of the small cut on the back of her head. She scrunched up her eyes, opened her mouth and let out the most awful of screams, the length of it causing her face to turn slightly blue as she pushed on, apparently not needing to let up for air. The doctor jumped back, horrified that such a tiny being could make such an ear-splitting sound, his entire career probably flashing in front of his eyes. I picked Eve up and held her to me, un-phased by her volume and colour, both being regular occurrences. The doctor ran for a nurse, and together they pressed a cold compress onto her head, the doctor apologising again and again. I brushed his apology off, telling him not to worry, it happened all the time; to be honest I was sorry my child was such a drama queen. If it had happened at home she would have gotten a quick kiss and been told to get on with it. John and I were outnumbered by almost feral babies from so early on in our parenting experience that we take the attitude of "what doesn't kill them makes them stronger" to quite an extreme level. Our children have taken to this mantra wholeheartedly, appearing to see everything in life as just one big climbing frame that they must explore. I try to tell myself that this is character building, but in reality I'm pretty sure I'm just raising circus performers and cat burglars. I tried to get the doctor to turn his attention back to my breathing test results. This was hard work, as he was much more interested in Eve's head, even offering to stitch it up for me. By this point the bleeding had all but stopped, and I told him I was sure it would be fine, it looked very superficial. He didn't take his eyes of her when I asked him for his opinion on my lung function, and vaguely made some non-specific comment about it. But he seemed to have lost his nerve and excused himself to go and find out what the consultant thought. We waited, a nurse now sitting with me and playing with the other two whilst I cuddled Eve, clearly trying not to laugh. Eve was absolutely fine. She stopped crying the second the doctor had left, and busied herself playing peek-a-boo with the patient in the next bed. Sometime later the doctor returned, and again went straight to Eve, who predictably began bawling reflexively the second he arrived on the ward, her eyes completely dry. He performed a complete examination of her, checking her pupils, her reflexes and carefully wiping her head with an alcohol wipe. She shrieked, but it was clearly just for show, the cut was tiny, obviously shallow and the small lump it had raised was already shrinking. She was completely fine. Satisfied, the doctor offered yet more apologies and walked off as fast as he could without actually running. I called after him, and he stopped dead, then slowly turned, a smile fixed to his face. Awkwardly I asked him what the consultant had said about my lung function and whether or not I needed to continue with my extra antibiotics. Flustered, he quickly relayed her message, and then turned and sped from the day unit, clearly desperate to be away from the crazy lady and her terrifying offspring. His departure was so speedy I didn't even have time to apologise to him again, and so turned and proffered my apologies to the nurses instead. "Don't worry, dear," the ward sister grinned wickedly. "WE'VE had a FANTASTIC time!" The nurses all grinned, nodding in agreeance and we left, the children happily waving to them and all the smiling patients. We probably had cheered their day up– the sight of me chasing my miscreant children round the ward, followed by the spectacle of a baby blatantly bullying a young doctor was probably a welcome relief from the boredom of the hospital for these patients. But I'm sure that night the poor doctor probably sat down and imbibed at least one alcoholic beverage.

The only time that I have completely overstepped the line and made a huge mistake with a hospital appointment was when I brought them with me not long after the girls had finished potty training. It could be argued that bringing three unruly children to any hospital appointment is a mistake, but there's not really much I can do about that. Potty training, for us, was a challenge. It seems to me that most parents struggle to know when the right time for potty training is. They agonise over when to pick the right moment to introduce it; neither too early nor too late. We didn't have this problem. In the January 4 months before his third birthday, Ben decided suddenly he no longer required nappies and wanted to use a potty. This was brilliant and after 4 days with minimal accidents we were done. We clapped ourselves on the back at how brilliant our parenting was and made the unbelievably ludicrous decision to buy a puppy to replace our deceased dog, reasoning it would be nice for the children to grow up with a dog around, and that with just two in nappies now would be the best time, everything suddenly feeling so much easier. Although as a springer spaniel Captain Dog (name courtesy of our nearly three-year-old son) should only be a small to medium sized dog his initially tiny frame was misleading, and all too soon he became a ridiculously humungous 27 kg of pure muscle. He's still growing, but hopefully he'll stop before he reaches horse proportions. Of course, pride always comes before a fall, and two weeks after the puppy arrived, the girls decided that they too could be free of nappies and do their business all over the house just like their new furry friend did. Unfortunately, they had barely any language and therefore couldn't communicate when they needed the toilet. Although only 16 months, my girls were (and still are) deeply determined, and I spent nearly a month trying to force them back into nappies before admitting defeat. They were sneaky and speedy, taking their nappies off and hiding them behind sofas, under the table and down the backs of their cots, then pulling their trousers back up so I didn't know they weren't wearing them until I stepped in a puddle or smelt a suspicious odour. After a few months of poo filled hell, my sanity barely intact, we'd finally made enough of a break through to call them potty trained.

For those painful months I managed to force the girls into nappies for my hospital appointments. I spent the whole time we were there watching them like a hawk for any bids for nappy freedom, but all went well. Once they'd finally trained, however, I bit the bullet and brought them along without nappies, instead slipping two potties into the bottom of their buggy. I did briefly consider leaving them with a friend instead, but I like my friends, and felt that leaving barely potty-trained twins with anyone was hardly conducive to a long-lasting friendship. We arrived at the appointment and settled into our clinic room as normal. Within a few minutes the girls decided they would try out the potties in this exciting new location. I was surprised they needed them so soon, but got them out anyway. Wees done, I realised too late that cross infection rules meant that I couldn't leave the room, and therefore had no way of emptying them. I wasn't too worried as they weren't big wees, and put them out of the way under my chair. Not to be out done, Ben also decided to use one. The respiratory therapist arrived whilst he was still sat on it. He looked slightly surprised to find a small boy sitting on a potty in the middle of the room, but took it in his stride. I began to do my breathing tests. Half way through my second blow Ben stood up behind the man and proudly tipped the potty forwards towards the man's head to show me his poo. I spluttered, ruining the test, and the man asked if I was ok. I didn't want to alarm him by telling him he'd almost become the victim of a callous poo attack, so I just said I was fine. After a couple more blows he was satisfied at the results and left as quickly as he could, the air in the small room already cloying. Ben had done another poo in the other potty, and I was stuck with both potties and a good hour at least of appointment to go. It's worth mentioning at this point that we were in the middle of a very hot, very long-lasting heat wave, and that the windows in the clinic rooms barely open. To make matters worse both the girls decided to add more wees in to the already rather full potties. The dietitian arrived, told me my weight seemed fine and left without even sitting down, in the quickest dietitian appointment I've ever had in 24 years of CF appointments. I had been going to ask her if there was anywhere I could sneak off too to empty the offending articles, but she'd gone so fast I didn't get the chance. Another three wees and a cheeky poo appeared (to this day I don't know how they were so prolific, I swear they joined forces and did it just to spite me) and I began to sweat, even briefly contemplating surreptitiously tipping them out of the window into the car park. Common sense prevailed and I realised this would be disgusting, and probably a slight infection control issue. The physio came in and almost held her nose, her questions quick and nasally. Fortunately, she seemed to find the whole thing amusing. I was too stressed to see the funny side by this point, especially as she could leave (again remarkably quickly) whereas I was trapped. By the time the doctor appeared we were at 14 wees and 4 poos, and the potties had reached absolute capacity. He didn't say much and I kept my answers to questions as succinct as possible. He then vanished off at pace, the appointment finally concluded. I breathed a shallow sigh of relief, before realising I now had to exit the building carrying a bag of toys, pushing a double buggy, holding a toddler's hand

and somehow balancing two precariously full potties. I made it, painfully slowly, through the nearly empty waiting area but was briefly thwarted by the double doors to the main corridor. Fortunately, a CF consultant was coming the other way. He opened the door and looked at me, taking in my ridiculous situation with a slightly disbelieving expression, then asked if he could help in any way. Almost crying with relief, I asked where to empty the potties as I hadn't been able to due to cross infection risks. He pointed to the loo down the corridor and quietly said I could probably just nip there in future if I ever got stuck again. All in all, it was the most stressful, most mortifying, but least time consuming appointment I've ever had.

-9-

THE END

When I was little, my parents told me I took my pills to help make me live longer. This, of course, was true, but I took it to mean that my life would be extended beyond normal limits. I used to proudly boast to my fellow primary school pupils that my pills gave me super powers, and that with them I would be living way into my hundreds. I spent a happy couple of years informing other children of this whenever they mentioned either my tablets or my cough. Fortunately, my boasts eventually reached the ears of my school teachers, who, probably somewhat horrified, passed this information onto my poor parents. As a result, my mother, on the drive home from one of my regular clinic appointments, had the difficult task of disabusing me of this wild theory. I remember very clearly how she cleared her throat awkwardly before asking if I knew what would happen because of my CF. I told her "nothing, I'm just going to take pills forever." The 1997 Blue Peter appeal had already taught me that CF was incurable, a fact that I pedalled happily to anyone who would listen. I knew what it meant in theory, but I was mostly just saying it for the kudos of using a big word, and to see the look on a grown-up's face when I said it. Mum was driving, so she didn't really look at me, but I could see her gripping the steering wheel slightly tighter. "It will stop you living as long as most people do." I was a bit taken aback, but simply asked how long I would live. "Probably until you're nearly 50," she said. "Oh. A long time then," I remember saying lightly, and we drove the rest of the way in silence. The truth was that I felt a little disappointed I would never become the World's Oldest Woman, a target I'd set myself as soon as I'd heard my pills were helping me live, but other than that I was fine. After all, to a 9-year-old, 50 seems a very long way away.

The following Monday, at the start of morning break time, I went to my teacher and asked him how old he was. He told me this was a rude question, but I persisted and asked if he was more than 50. He replied that he was, and asked why I wanted to know. "Because I'm not going to be as old as you," I replied. "My Mum says I'm going to die before then." My poor teacher looked somewhat taken aback, and I turned and skipped off, bunches swinging, to play Spice Girls. I remember this incident vividly, because about five minutes later, whilst my friends and I perfected our "Wannabe" dance, I caught sight of him watching me through the class room window. The expression on his face told me straight away that death wasn't something I should really be talking about, and I tried to put it out of my mind.

Although my mother and I never discussed it again, the knowledge that I was living with a disease that would eventually kill me did weigh quite heavily on me for a long time. Even on that short journey home from the hospital I began to realise that 50 wasn't actually that old. After all, my grandparents were all still very active (my paternal grandparents extremely so – on retirement they took up mountaineering and world travelling, and were always off on another adventure) and yet they were all quite a way over 50.

As I entered my teenage years this information resurfaced unexpectedly. I became obsessed with telling friends at school (or anyone who mentioned my cough) that CF was a terrible illness that killed people, but not me. I had a special, mild kind I said, in my wisest 12-year-old voice, and therefore would not be dying young. Although death is a taboo subject amongst adults, amongst children it's fair game to discuss. I don't believe any of my classmates ever gave their own death a second thought, and therefore they were happy to chat about it openly whenever I brought it up. Indeed, it almost became a joke to some. I remember a P.E. lesson in year 8 where we had to do the dreaded bleep test. I was one of the last two running the length of the sports hall between endless, quickening bleeps, when a defeated classmate called out "It's alright for Abi, she's motivated. Not running enough won't kill us!" The P.E teacher was horrified, but we all laughed and the other girl dropped out with a "good point" shrug.

As I've grown up past being a school girl, conversations about death have become less and less frequent. Generally, my CF comes up within the first few times of meeting someone – usually through a sympathetic mention of my cough. I make no secret of it and will happily tell anyone that I have it, but on average it takes a further 6 months before a new friend or acquaintance asks a bit more about it, and the obvious question of life expectancy is usually avoided for a further two years. Eventually the person plucks up the courage to ask me if my CF will kill me. I suspect they know the answer already from google, but can't quite believe a person who looks so normal on the outside can be so messed up within. I used to just say "yes" and watch them flounder in the silence, but I soon realised this was mean and so now say "yes, but hopefully not for a long time." I then give some statistics, but emphasise that every person is different. The response to this information is almost invariably "Oh! I'm so sorry," and is followed almost instantly by some sort of innocuous comment about the weather. Obviously, I don't enjoy these conversations, but the pattern and unapologetic British-ness of them is something I find quietly amusing.

In hindsight, I think talking about death early on was actually a very good thing. I've read a lot about patients who fight against their CF and often become non-compliant with their meds, especially in their teenage years. I won't pretend I'm perfect, and no-one could consistently take all the medication we have, always do their physio twice a day, swallow all the supplements, eat all the food and do all the exercise required without some off periods, especially not whilst living a normal life, attending normal school/college/university, holding down a job and/or raising a family. (And my medication load is tiny in comparison to most patients!) But I do believe that a lot of people get too depressed taking their meds because they are a daily reminder of what's going on in their bodies, and what's coming in the future. I wonder whether perhaps some CF patients aren't made aware of the fact that they are dying young enough for it to become normal before the naturally rebellious teenage years happen, and therefore, understandably, they see their medications and treatments as an imposition on their short lives, rather than as enablers of a slightly longer one. The horrible truth is that no matter how hard you work at it, CF will always win. Every infection will leave that little bit more damage. The secretions slowly inflame the lungs and digestive system more and more until there's nothing that can be done. There is no cure, and all the treatments are just slowing the inevitable.

As a child who grew up through the age of internet, I was able to gather large amounts of detailed information about my condition without having any adult vet it. My mother always told people not to google CF, because every case is different, and the internet will only show the worst. Not to research CF too much was the advice my paediatric consultant had given my parents, probably to stop them falling into a deep pit of depression. I had carefully listened to this advice, but when I had just turned 13 I decided to take things into my own hands. I skipped my lunch at school and went to the library. I sat at one of the three computers; the one furthest away from the librarian's desk, and guiltily typed "cystic fibrosis" into the search engine, opening Pandora's box on the screen in front of me. I began with basic information that I already knew, but soon delved into terrifying, incomprehensible articles. I read and read and read, using the whole hour, two tabs open on the browser; a medical journal and a dictionary. The more I read, the more obvious it became that hope would not be fluttering out. I logged in and read every lunch time that week, and continued to do so periodically throughout my time at secondary school. Indeed, my most harrowing experience was reading a scholarly article on a computer in the school library whilst "doing my English Coursework" after school. The article explored how a CF team dealt with patient deaths, how to improve patient, family and staff experiences and how to facilitate "good" deaths. Obviously, this was not appropriate reading for a 15-year-old, but at least I was informed, and, therefore, became more and more determined to stave off the worst. As well as learning about how CF deaths occurred, obsessively reading all the gritty details in every medical journal I could find it referenced in, I quickly discovered that my mother's estimate of my life expectancy was in fact just that. A vague, rather optimistic, estimate. Although living to 50 (or even, in rare cases, beyond) is possible, there is a high chance of a much earlier demise.

Now as a person with good lung function (for a person with CF!) fluctuating but generally not desperately low weight and good overall health, thinking about death in my 20s could seem melodramatic and unnecessarily morbid. However, the average age of death for a CF patient is actually 29-35, and in 2017 eighty-two of the one hundred and thirty-two people who died of CF were under the age of 35. That's 62%. Too many people are dying young with CF. Actually, so young that my whole understanding of age in the CF community is askew compared to normal life. I think of CF patients in their 30s, and the few in the 40s and above as "old". In fact, when I researched the latest death statistics for this book I read that in theory with all the advances in medication and treatments that have taken place since the 1990s it is believed that over half of the patients born in the nineties and later, like I was, could reach 41 or above. This is of course a projected estimate as we're all still only 29 and under, but it is a lot more promising than the late teens expectancy my parents were given when I was first diagnosed. On reading this I nearly stopped writing. After all, why raise awareness for something that's practically cured? And then I realised that really, 41 isn't that old at all. Strangely I don't put myself in either camp (I'm sure a psychologist would label that as 'denial'), and I hope to be as old as possible when I finally go. But at the same time, I can't bring myself to take out a pension, as statistically it's unlikely that that I'll ever draw on it.

Although I am acutely aware that most die younger, the brief conversation with my mother has stuck with me, and I mentally think of 50 as being my cut off point. 50 is still a long way away for me, but it feels a lot closer than it did almost 20 years ago in my Mother's car. Indeed, some of my own friends have turned, or are turning, 50. It feels strange for people I spend time with to reach a number I myself have put such an emphasis on. I'm happy (obviously!) for friends when they reach the milestone but it's slightly marred with a selfish resentment that they have crossed over into an age that I am unlikely reach. As a child, I thought people in their 50s were probably OAPs. Now when I hear about someone without CF who has died in their 50s, their youth is the biggest tragedy that people mourn. To quote a friend who recently turned 50: "I could have half of my life left!" I must here state, categorically, that there are a minority of people with CF who have passed the age of

50, and, in theory, there is no reason why I (or any other CF patient) can't. I fully intend to live a very long life, reaching way beyond this milestone. However, for every person over 50, there are a lot who die in their 20s or even younger, and ambition cannot always be realised.

Cystic fibrosis deaths are, like I suppose all deaths, deeply unpleasant. This is partially because the patient is usually a young adult, which means that they are generally strong enough for the final stage to drag on, especially when there is the possibility of reprieve before the end in the form of a transplant, and so full palliative care is not actively undertaken for every patient. It is also partially because in most cases the patient essentially drowns in their own lungs. I understand that this is horrible to watch, and very painful to experience. In 95% of cases the patient is overcome with infection, and so passes away. The lungs are often so damaged by recurrent, long lasting infections, so full of mucus and so scarred, that they can't get the oxygen in fast enough and therefore the body shuts down. This final stage is awful, but it is important to remember that people with CF don't just float happily through life, then suddenly drop dead when they reach the end of their allotted time. There is not completely healthy or dying. Instead they go through life, living normal lives like mine, constantly battling chronic infections, getting knocked down by them and having to pick themselves up again and again, whilst in the background their organs are slowly blocking up. Eventually the fight becomes too much and they finally keel over with the exhaustion of it all.

Now CF death can be the result of a slow decline, but it can also be very sudden. Every new infection has the potential to be "the one" although CF teams are very quick to start patients on treatments before infections really take hold. Every patient will react differently to every infection. All people are intrinsically different, and therefore any new infection might just be that little too much for a person's immune system. Old, deep rooted infections can also flare up at any time, just to make life that little bit less certain. I personally have never been anywhere near dying from my CF, and hopefully won't be for a long time to come, but that doesn't mean I don't sometimes think about it.

In recent years, becoming a mother myself has made me apprehensive about my own mortality. As Ben and the girls are getting older it is becoming more and more necessary to explain things to them. My own parents never lied to me about my health, and I won't do it to my own children. Although explaining a life limiting genetic condition to a three-year-old and twin two year olds sounds like a thankless and somewhat foolish task, I feel it is important for the children to grow up knowing what's going on and seeing it as normal, however abnormal it may be. After all, I'm always popping pills around them, inhaling nebs, vanishing off to hospital appointments or stays, and generally coughing so they aren't exactly hidden from it all. They're also observant children who ask a lot of questions, and are often remarkably astute. This is partially why I bring them with me to hospital appointments. I want them to know the hospital and my CF team, so that as time goes on and I have to spend more and more time there they won't be thrust into something they know nothing about, with people they've never met. This attitude, however, has already led to some difficult conversations

When Ben was not quite two and a half our beloved dog Rosie had an horrific accident late one August night. John had taken her out for a walk and she somehow impaled herself on a branch. John raced home with her and shouted up to me as I was reading Ben's bedtime story that Rosie was poorly and I needed to come quickly. I said a quick goodnight to Ben and came downstairs. To cut a long story short, we had her put down at midnight that night. The next day I had to explain to Ben that his best friend Rosie was dead and would not be returning. As expected, Ben took it very badly. For weeks he lay around crying, unable to come to terms with her loss. But as the weeks of tears went on, it became apparent that he was mourning for more than just the loss of his four-legged friend. He became terrified of being "poorly" and I carefully explained to him, on more than one occasion, that "being poorly" didn't always mean that someone died. But his innocence had been shattered. He understood what death was and felt it keenly. A month later, on the way home from attending another hospital appointment with me, he asked the question I'd been dreading. "Mummy, are you poorly?" Sort of, I explained, but the doctors and my tablets were all working hard to keep me well. He was silent for a while, but then popped out the question I'd been dreading. "Mummy, will you die?" This was challenging. The truthful answer is always the best, but Ben wasn't even three. But if I lied, and then something did go wrong, would he always remember that I'd lied to him? So, I told the truth, and told him that yes, I would die, but hopefully not for a very long time. This seemed to satisfy him and I thought he'd forget about it. Two weeks later, however, on the way home from toddler group we passed through the village churchyard. Ben, chubby hand holding mine as I pushed his baby sisters in their buggy, suddenly looked up at me and said, "Daddy says dead people go here. People bring flowers. I'll bring flowers when you're too poorly Mummy. Daddy will help me." I didn't really know what to say, so we moved on. But in that moment, I hated CF more than I ever had before.

I sometimes worry that I have introduced the concept of death too early for the children. But perhaps this is actually a silly worry caused by a taboo we've created as a society. As a society, we just do not talk about death. We are not particularly exposed to it, and therefore we don't think about it, or consider that it will happen to us. We all know someone who, when faced with the death of an elderly relative, has expressed not just grief at their passing, but anger that doctors didn't do more. I have a friend who often works in intensive care, and the hardest part of her job is explaining to family members that nothing more can be done for their loved one. Naturally this is hard, but it is the anger that she finds most difficult, and her worst stories are always of attempting to resuscitate desperately ill, extremely elderly people, however hopeless their case is. Society seems to believe that doctors are magicians, and that they are able to halt death no matter how ill, or how damaged, a person is. Medicine will never be that good, and there will always be things that cannot be fixed. Death is the most certain part of life, and perhaps if we all took stock and thought about this hard truth every once in a while, then maybe, just maybe, we would all be that little bit happier with our lot.

Despite this keen realisation, I try not to think too much about the future anymore, and prefer to enjoy every day as it comes. Mostly this works well, but every now and again a slight feeling of panic sets in (usually around my birthday) and I spend a few days feeling melancholic. A strong appreciation of my own inevitable death could lead me to live an understandably rather depressed life, but so many people with CF are not as fortunate as me and I'm always conscious that things are (so far!) going pretty well for me. My CF is a big part of my life, and has been for so long, that I don't really think about it. Instead I see it as a sideshow to the main event, although it would be impossible for it not to be an ever-present goblin in the corner of every room. The physical evidence takes up shelves in my kitchen, a sharps bin sits in my living room and the draining rack is never free of nebuliser parts. My personal appearance, however normal I may look on first glance, is also a sign – skinny (sometimes frighteningly so) and frequently coughing. And, finally, my diary is run around pharmacy trips, repeat prescription phone calls, homecare delivery slots, hospital stays and, of course, clinic appointments.

The latter are very, very regular and friends who aren't chronically ill often mention how frequent my appointments are, regularly commenting that I see my doctors so frequently we must be "good friends". This is definitely not the case, but it does cause me to reflect on how weird my relationship with my CF team is. They know everything about me, everything that has happened in my adult life and everything medical that has happened to me since I was diagnosed at the age of four. They know my husband, my children. They've supported me through two pregnancies, a handful of minor operations and increasingly frequent hospital stays. They've helped me when treatments have made me sick, and one consultant once sat and comforted me when I cried at needing my first lot of IVs. For goodness sake, they even know all the latest gossip about my bowel movements. Conversely, I know nothing about them. I know their names, and a few have vaguely mentioned their own children. I think one of them might have some cats. And that's it. They are a huge part of my life; since moving my care to my current hospital at the age of 21 I've spent approximately 1610 hours of the last 8 years of my life around them, yet they remain almost anonymous. Although from an external perspective this may seem cold, I don't see this as a bad thing. After all the doctors, nurses, physios, dietitians and pharmacists who make up a CF team are always very busy looking after a lot of patients, the vast majority of whom will die at some point during their career. It must be a strange job to spend so much time seeing and helping the same patients again and again, watching their personal lives unfold, whilst knowing each and every one of them is slowly (or indeed quickly) travelling towards an untimely death. From my own small experiences of being a shoulder to cry on for my friends who are doctors and nurses when they lose a slightly more long-term patient or are present for a particularly difficult death, I can only imagine what the psychological toll of caring for patients for their whole adult life only to watch them die young anyway must be. Self-preservation and common sense must force a clinical air on to everything. I'm happy about this – I like everyone in the CF team, but I don't want to be too friendly with people, however nice, who want to know about my poo, and will eventually care for me as I die.

As horrible as all this is, I'm not actually afraid of dying. Naturally when the time comes I'm sure I will be, but for now I've made my peace with it. Death is an unavoidable part of cystic fibrosis, a fact I came to an acceptance of in my teenage years, after first spending an inordinate amount of time obsessively pouring over every article about CF I could find in every medical journal I could locate online, desperately trying to find out how to cheat my way out of my situation, whilst crying about it silently at night. The more I read, the more I realised this wasn't an option, and I began to accept it, reminding myself that death comes to everyone, and no one can really know when the proverbial bus will hit them. It's not the thought of death that scares me, but the time before. The bit in between living a normal life and finally dying, when my CF will have to become the main focus in my life, with treatments and hospital stays filling more time than the normal things of life take. I don't want my children to think of me as their "poorly Mummy", or my husband to have to slow down work because I'm too ill to take care of the house, the children and myself. Hopefully I'm a long time from that, but unfortunately there is no way of stopping decline in CF, and therefore this is a sure and certain future. So far, I have managed to keep my life in two distinct boxes; normal life and CF life. Recently, however, it has felt as though the lines are beginning to blur a little. My CF team and I may be working as hard as possible to slow this decline, but however hard I step on the brake the car continues to creep forwards. At some point it will gain momentum, and eventually there will be very little I can do to stop it. I can't complain though - I'm 28 and, so far, I have been very lucky.

-10-

THE FUTURE

Now we're at the final chapter, you could be forgiven for thinking that this book will end on a deeply depressing note. As things currently stand I would probably be forced to end with some hideously "inspirational" quotes about making lemonade and learning to dance in the rain, or perhaps just talk about how much I've learned on my "journey", until the weight of all the quasi-positivity causes you to vomit all over the page. But fear not.

There is no denying that cystic fibrosis is a horrible, life limiting, multi system condition that slowly and painfully takes from the sufferer every ability to breathe, eat and eventually live. I may only be mildly affected, but it still takes a lot of time and effort to manage, and sooner or later it will catch up with me. The vast majority of the other people who suffer from it are not as lucky as me, and are often very ill from very young. But don't worry, there's no need to brace yourself, because the reality is that there has recently been a huge shift in the way that cystic fibrosis is treated. This has brought hope, and a much better quality of life, to many.

Up until now every pill and treatment that has been given to and used by a CF patient has treated symptoms and complications of the condition. New drugs have been developed that get to the root of the problem, treating the cause thus lessening the symptoms and therefore the complications. The latest drug, Orkambi, is so good that it's been nicknamed 'the wonder drug' and the next drug, the Triple (or Trikafta), is looking even better.

To understand how these drugs work we need to go back to the very basics of CF, and appreciate what's actually going wrong. Cystic fibrosis, for all of its complicated associated problems, is actually very simple and starts with one tiny fault in the CF gene. The CF gene is located in the brain (nucleus) of the epithelial cell, and is responsible for telling the cell to produce CFTR proteins. Everyone has two CF genes, but people with cystic fibrosis have a tiny fault in both of their CF genes, which means the CFTR proteins the epithelial cell makes are faulty, and so cystic fibrosis occurs.

Now the CFTR protein has one simple but highly important job. It is made in the cell and travels to the wall of the cell where it pushes through and acts like a tunnel, allowing chloride to pass out of the cell and into the airways (or intestine/pancreas etc.) The chloride then mixes with the mucus, pulling water out of the cell and allowing the cilia (hairs) on the external walls of the cells to waft the now loosened mucus away and out.

In cystic fibrosis, there is a fault in the gene. The gene is like an instruction manual, and in cystic fibrosis there is a mistake on the page. In a normal person, the cell reads the instructions and makes the protein. But in cystic fibrosis the instructions are wrong and therefore the cell makes a faulty protein (or in some cases just don't make one at all.) This happens again and again as the cell cannot understand that there is a fault. As a result, the chloride does not pass out of the cell and so the balance of salt and water is wrong, causing the mucus on the other side of the cell in the tubes to be stickier and therefore much harder to shift.

Because the tiny fault in the CF gene instruction manual is just one typo, it can be anywhere on the page. At the moment scientists have identified 2000 different faults. Some typos (or faults) are more common than others, and one called DeltaF508 is the most common fault. Due to the wide number of possible faults there are a few different things that can happen during the production of the CFTR protein and as a result there is quite a range of severity to the disease. Some people are unable to make CFTR proteins at all, whereas some make them and they travel to the cell wall, but aren't as effective at passing the chloride out as they should be. In addition to this the protein tube has a gate in it, which opens and closes to let the chloride ions out. This is often stuck, or does not open anywhere near enough to let the chloride out. The most common fault, caused by the DeltaF508 gene, is for the CFTR protein to be made flat but then not folded round into a tube shape. This means that if it does make it to the wall of the cell it cannot pass out any chloride. Personally, I have one DeltaF508 gene and one gene (IF507) that causes minimal function. Although there are degrees of severity to the disease because of this, additional factors (such as infections, treatment regimes, additional health problems, natural immune system strength etc.) pay such a huge part that there isn't really good and bad CF, and when push comes to shove all of us will die from it anyway. Some people might just have things weighted a little more heavily against them.

The new drugs act directly on the CFTR protein, thus dealing with the problem at it's very core. Orkambi is a drug for people with two copies of the most common mutation of the CF gene, DeltaF508. This drug is made of two drugs called lumacaftor and ivacaftor. Lumacaftor helps the protein bend round into a tube, thus allowing it to push through the wall of the cell. Ivacaftor helps the gate in the tube open up more frequently, so the chloride ions can pass out and mix with the mucus, making it less sticky, therefore allowing the cilia to actually do their job. This is, quite frankly, genius. It is not a cure, but it will make a huge difference to the life of a patient with CF.

Orkambi will improve the situation for many patients, but it is the next drug, the Triple, that we are really looking forward to. The Triple is a combination of three new drugs (tezacaftor, elexacaftor and ivacaftor) and the recently released data from the latest clinical trial demonstrated a 10% increase in the lung function of patients on the trial in just 4 weeks. It is for the approximately 90% of CF patients who have either two copies of the DeltaF508 gene, (known as "double deltas") or who have one DeltaF508 and one other. This includes myself. Before too long CF patients could sit down and take a drug every day that will help us manage our mucus production, thus helping us shift the nasty stuff out of our lungs, resulting in improved lung function, fewer lung infections and therefore less hospital stays and a better quality of life. It will also help with mucus production elsewhere in the body, although this much-needed benefit is slightly harder to measure. Whilst these drugs and their effects are fantastic for an adult, a lot of long lasting damage has already been caused. They are undeniably brilliant for adults, but imagine giving them to a child. A child with lungs relatively undamaged by infection, and a gut yet to be damaged by the mucus build up. These drugs are not perfect. They will not cure a person, and CF will still affect them, but it will not be to the same extent. We are living in truly exciting times, and the future is looking bright.

But there's a problem.

Orkambi, although 4 years old, is not available in the UK on the NHS. It's considered too expensive. Now £104,000 a year is a lot of money, I won't deny that. But at the same time, this drug didn't happen overnight. 18 years of hard work and investment have gone into Orkambi, and time, money and effort are still going in to the Triple and further projects. The company who makes them, Vertex Pharmaceuticals, has pledged to continue working on finding a cure for CF, and needs the money to do this. The amount of money this sort of research takes is truly mind blowing, and the cost of the drugs unfortunately have to reflect this in order to recoup investment whilst moving forwards. On top of this if these drugs were for an illness such as cancer, which affects the lives of a lot more patients, the cost per drug would be smaller as more drugs would be sold. Unfortunately, CF is commonly rare. Although it is the most common life limiting genetic disease, in the UK there are only about 10,000 of us living with it, and only about 45% of those are double deltas. This means that the high development costs have to be split between not very many people.

In the past 4 years, I have heard many an argument put forwards against Orkambi. The most common of which are it's too expensive, it's not effective enough and worst, and most shockingly, of all: CF patients will still die younger anyway, so what's the point? On the face of it, these arguments seem reasonable. But are they really?

Firstly, the argument that CF patients will eventually die anyway is a bizarre one. It is true that Orkambi and the Triple are not cures, and CF patients will still be prone to infections, but it will be much more manageable, and therefore life expectancy will dramatically increase. Indeed, a consultant at a leading London Hospital recently wrote that he estimates the Triple could add as much as 27 years to a person's life. When life expectancy is only twenty-nine, 27 years is another lifetime on top. Yes, of course CF patients will still die younger, but it will buy us a lot more time. Short lives will considerably lengthen. Benjamin Franklin reportedly said, "in this world nothing can be said to be certain, except death and taxes." All people will eventually die, and withholding medical treatment because of this fact is ludicrous. If we follow this through to its logical conclusion we should stop giving anyone any medical help. Hospitals should shut and medical professionals get different jobs to help our new totalitarian state. Undertaking perhaps. It may seem that this argument against Orkambi is so odd that it's not worth giving time too, but worryingly I've had it said to my face on more than one occasion.

Often when I am asked about Orkambi, it comes hand in hand with questions about transplant. Lung transplants (and pancreas and sometimes liver transplants) are used in CF as a way to stave off the worst. Replacing damaged lungs with lungs that aren't scarred from years of infections and don't have epithelial cells with faulty genes in is good. But they aren't a cure. The cystic fibrosis is still everywhere else in the body, although the lungs may now be free. Sometimes people look at me and ask why I don't just go and get a new pair of lungs. In theory, this sounds a wonderful idea, although it does perhaps show how little awareness there is of the other aspects of CF. But transplants are not simple. Aside from lungs not being available freely, the operation is hugely traumatic and not always survivable. The recovery is hard, and from the moment the new lungs are put in there is the chance that the body will reject them. Eventually they will be rejected, 50% of the time within the first 5 years, but in the meantime copious amounts of expensive medication have to be taken to stop this. Transplants are incredible, and anyone who has had one has been through more than anyone who hasn't, like myself, can imagine. But they are not the best solution, and the operation and follow up life-long medical care are considerably more expensive than Orkambi. Not everyone is suitable for a transplant, and not everyone would want one.

Secondly, people argue that Orkambi is not actually effective enough to warrant its cost. In fairness, the effectiveness of Orkambi is difficult to measure fully. No, it doesn't cure. But what it does is amazing, and in years to come we will see a vast improvement in life expectancy because of it. Drugs that are tackling the route of the problem cannot give instantaneous effects. Instead the effects are cumulative, but the initial signs are more than promising. It has so far been reported that patients on Orkambi are suffering 30-39% less exacerbations, or infection flare ups. This means a lot less hospital time, and a lot less additional antibiotics, as well as a better quality of life. Doctors who are treating patients now on Orkambi say that they see a huge difference in the morbidity (signs of serious illness) that the patient has. Patients are looking better, which is a sign that the drug is doing a lot on the inside. Vertex aren't resting on their laurels, and doctors are also still working on researching CF. The Triple is the next drug along, and has been developed by building upon the learnings from Orkambi. A cure may one day be possible, but without laying the foundations now by using these remarkable drugs and gaining the financial resources from them I do not see how a cure could ever be reached.

These new drugs will benefit 90% of the World CF population, begging the obvious question: what about the other 10%? These highly unfortunate people have sadly got a class of mutations that actually stop the

201

epithelial cell from producing any CFTR protein at all, rather than there being a problem with the protein once it has been made. Obviously, this is a very different problem, even though the results may be the same. This means that the current set of new drugs cannot help them, and they are stuck waiting and hoping for their chance. Vertex is looking into this, and are trying to fix this problem as well. But this will come at a price, as sadly no research can be done for free, and no drug is chanced upon in a scientist's first attempt. (Even Fleming didn't know exactly what he had, and penicillin was passed on to a team of other scientists who took a further 13 years to take it from initial findings to mass production.) We owe it to the 10% to make the money available for this life changing research, and this will only come through the money paid for the medications that have already been made.

Finally, yes, Orkambi is expensive. I have listed the reasons why Vertex claims they need so much money for it above. However, the statement that it is TOO expensive to justify giving it needs to have an additional level of scrutiny put to it. Currently, CF patients take up a large amount of NHS resources. We're heavy prescription drug users, we fill hospital beds for weeks or months at a time, we require huge amounts of attention from specialist teams and I dread to think what the cost of all the food hospitals shove at us is. In other words, we're expensive. All of the care and attention even someone as well as myself gets costs a lot of money. My CF nurse told me last year that it's not uncommon for CF patients to have over £100,000 in just IV drugs a year. That doesn't include non-IV antibiotics, steroids, enzymes, specially high vitamins, antacids, anti-sickness, inhalers, bronchodilators, liver medications, nasal sprays, feeding tubes, supplements, insulin, calcium, oxygen, needles… the list could go on. Just one of my nebulisers (Dornase Alfa) costs £500 per month. We also take the time of doctors, surgeons, dietitians, physios, pharmacists, specialist nurses, social workers, psychologists, microbiologists. And that's just the higher paid staff. We also take the time of hospital cleaners, housekeepers, HCAs. Although all these people would still be needed even if we spent less time hanging around in hospitals coughing gunk everywhere, they would all be able to focus on other patients more. The NHS is pouring money into us, but not looking at its long-term investment. Those who have received Orkambi in other countries have been shown to have considerably less exacerbations and therefore less hospital time and less need for IVs, as well as less need for extra medication. If Orkambi and the Triple were given then CF patients would actually be considerably cheaper. This doesn't even take into account the patients who are currently too ill to work who could go back into employment and therefore pay into the system, rather than being forced simply to take in the form of benefits.

Unfortunately, the governing body that controls what drugs the NHS will pay for (NICE) does not see it this way. These new drugs are so beyond anything anyone has seen before they are not able to measure how wonderful they are. Although anecdotal evidence is highly promising, it will take more time for the evidence from other countries to stack up so that the benefit is undeniable in every way. This is time that CF patients do not have. Every day we wait, we have more mucus, more infections, more damage. More die waiting.

Orkambi has been given on compassionate grounds to some of the most ill patients in the UK, and in many of these cases has been life changing for those who have received it. But this is not enough. The damage has been done, and although the patient experiences a much greater quality of life, if they had received the drug before they were so ill they would be seeing a much more long-term benefit. For most people CF is slowly eking away at them, but the tables can always turn, and damage done can't always be overcome. In most cases, Orkambi freezes the situation where it is, stopping the clock where things currently stand. The Triple actually actively improves it. Currently clinicians are like firefighters returning to a house again and again to put out fires, tipping their helmets to the match wielding arsonist on their way out. Logically they should be calling the police to whisk the nutter away, but a quirk in budget means the police force will only come out when the property is almost beyond saving. This, as you can appreciate, is beyond frustrating for both doctor and patient alike.

Imagine living daily with a serious disease, knowing that it could be hugely improved. Imagine waiting for years for this breakthrough, only to be told you can't have it. It's depressing, ridiculous and not even cost effective. The current stand-off between NICE and Vertex is causing anguish for CF patients, families, friends, medical staff. And it's just entered a fourth year.

Enough is enough. This is a scandal. Sadly, the average person on the street doesn't know about it, and horrifyingly most politicians seem not to care. Cystic fibrosis patients are young and a tiny, tiny minority of the population. We do not have the power to force change. Weak voices are weakening further, worn down with exhaustion and anguish. Not being able to get together to share our frustrations and demonstrate is proving a huge hindrance, and as a result the issue is being swept under the carpet.

So please, write to your MP. Ask them why they aren't pushing for NICE and Vertex to do a deal. Ask them to attend the parliamentary debates. Sign the online petitions. Email the health secretary. Tell your neighbour about the young people dying for breath, waiting for a relief they could already be having. Think about the babies who are being born with the chance to live normal lives, but who's insides are still being damaged by a mucus problem that could be hugely reduced. We need these drugs, and we need them now.

This scandal must stop.

AUTHOR'S NOTE

Thursday 24th October 2019 was a momentous day for the UK CF community. After a 4-year deadlock, NHS England and Vertex finally agreed to a deal allowing Orkambi and Symkevi to be given to all CF patients in the UK with the double delta CF gene.

Finally these CF patients have the chance to live better lives, with fewer hospital stays and fewer IV antibiotics courses. They will not be cured, but their illness will not have such cruel daily effects and hopefully they will have happier, fuller lives.

Most excitingly for me, this deal paves the way for future medications – particularly the Triple. I am still waiting for my precision treatment, my better life, but it is now almost within my grasp.

My hope for the future of CF is that CF patients living ordinary lives like mine (if not even better, healthier lives) will be the rule, and not the exception.

ACKNOWLEDGEMENTS

I wrote this book in a hospital room as an inpatient in a fit of frustration and rage at the unfairness of Orkambi and Symkevi not being available on the NHS. After 4 years of campaigning the CF community was still not getting the treatments we so desperately needed, and I was becoming increasingly conscious of how little awareness and understanding of the condition there is. My hope was that writing a book about what CF really is, and how it fills the life of even a mildly affected person, might help the cause. My thanks go to those who agreed that this was a good idea, and have encouraged me to publish it even now that Orkambi and Symkevi are available. Let's all hope that the Triple will not take so long.

Special thanks must go to Julia Nicholson for painstakingly picking through every chapter to check for both medical and grammatical errors.

Thankyou also to Elsa Milner, Rebecca Clare and James Thorpe for being willing to read my first full draft. Also thankyou to Michael Thorpe for your final read through.

Thankyou also to my parents, without whom this book could not have been written, for giving me such a strong foundation for my life.

Thankyou to my wonderful husband John for your support throughout our relationship, especially in this last, most difficult, year. Thankyou also for all the Calshakes you made me when I was editing, I am grateful for them all. Honest.

And finally, a big thankyou to all those who work in the NHS, whatever your role. But especially to my current CF team who are all hard working, deeply compassionate and have never once rolled their eyes in my presence at either mine or my children's madness. That in itself deserves a medal.

For further information about cystic fibrosis visit:

www.cysticfibrosis.org.uk
www.cff.org